Kept 12/2013

DATE DUE

JAN	0 4 2011		
AUG 2 2	2011		

APHASIA: SYMPTOMS, DIAGNOSIS AND TREATMENT

LANGUAGES AND LINGUISTICS SERIES

Critical Discourse Analysis: An Interdisciplinary Perspective
Thao Le, Quynh Le and Megan Short (Editors)
2009. ISBN 978-1-60741-320-2

Building Language Skills and Cultural Competencies in the Military
Edgar D. Swain (Editor)
2009. ISBN 978-1-60741-126-0

Second Languages: Teaching, Learning and Assessment
Ryan L. Jikal and Samantha A. Raner (Editors)
2009. ISBN 978-1-60692-661-1

Aphasia: Symptoms, Diagnosis and Treatment
Grigore Ibanescu and Serafim Pescariu (Editors)
2009. ISBN: 978-1-60741-288-5

LANGUAGES AND LINGUISTICS SERIES

APHASIA: SYMPTOMS, DIAGNOSIS AND TREATMENT

GRIGORE IBANESCU AND
SERAFIM PESCARIU
EDITORS

Nova Biomedical Books
New York

For permission to use material from this book please contact us:
Telephone 631-231-7269; Fax 631-231-8175
Web Site: http://www.novapublishers.com

NOTICE TO THE READER

The Publisher has taken reasonable care in the preparation of this book, but makes no expressed or implied warranty of any kind and assumes no responsibility for any errors or omissions. No liability is assumed for incidental or consequential damages in connection with or arising out of information contained in this book. The Publisher shall not be liable for any special, consequential, or exemplary damages resulting, in whole or in part, from the readers' use of, or reliance upon, this material.

Independent verification should be sought for any data, advice or recommendations contained in this book. In addition, no responsibility is assumed by the publisher for any injury and/or damage to persons or property arising from any methods, products, instructions, ideas or otherwise contained in this publication.

This publication is designed to provide accurate and authoritative information with regard to the subject matter covered herein. It is sold with the clear understanding that the Publisher is not engaged in rendering legal or any other professional services. If legal or any other expert assistance is required, the services of a competent person should be sought. FROM A DECLARATION OF PARTICIPANTS JOINTLY ADOPTED BY A COMMITTEE OF THE AMERICAN BAR ASSOCIATION AND A COMMITTEE OF PUBLISHERS.

Library of Congress Cataloging-in-Publication Data

Aphasia : symptoms, diagnosis and treatment / editors, Grigore Ibanescu and Serafim Pescariu.
    p. cm.
Includes index.
ISBN 978-1-60741-288-5 (hardcover)
1. Aphasia. I. Ibanescu, Grigore. II. Pescariu, Serafim.
RC425.A59 2009
616.85'52--dc22
                        2009031036

Published by Nova Science Publishers, Inc. ✦ *New York*

Contents

Preface

Aphasia is a language disorder in which there is an impairment (but not loss) of speech and of comprehension of speech. Depending on the area and extent of the damage, someone suffering from aphasia may be able to speak but not write, or vice versa, or display any of a wide variety of other deficiencies in language comprehension and production. This book will review grammatical world class processing by aphasic individuals and bilingual aphasia, each of which is essential to an understanding of the topic. This book will also examine the role of the right hemisphere for language processing and successful therapeutic interventions in aphasic patients. Furthermore, new findings for the understanding of neural processes involved in the recovery of language functions in aphasic subjects are discussed. This book also expands and improves upon the currently accepted methodology used in the diagnosis of dementia, particularly when aphasia is a core symptom. Finally, dual-route models and right-hemispheric accounts are examined to predict comprehension of figurative language in healthy speakers as well as in patients with language disorders.

Chapter I - This chapter will review two major areas in the aphasiology literature, (i) grammatical word class processing by aphasic individuals and (ii) bilingual aphasia, each of which is essential to an understanding of the topic. The first relates to *grammatical word class processing*, specifically that for *verbs* and *nouns*. This area is extremely important because word-finding difficulties for verbs and nouns are so common in aphasia. Also, the processing differences between verbs and nouns that occur at various levels of linguistic analysis: semantic, syntactic, morphological, and phonological will be highlighted. In addition, an overview of the major research studies that have specifically investigated verb-noun dissociations and the patterns of verb and noun impairments in aphasic syndromes is provided. Evidence from neuroimaging studies is also reviewed. The findings reported will be considered in relation to explanatory models locating the breakdown at either linguistic or neuroanatomical levels.

Furthermore, in this chapter, I will focus on grammatical word class breakdown in the context of bilingual aphasia. This section will highlight what little is known about how verbs and nouns are processed in bilingual patients due to the reliance on monolingual subjects in these studies. I will present up-to-date research available on *investigating grammatical word class distinctions* and, indeed, in different languages, in people with bilingual aphasia.

This focus is also significant for a theoretical understanding of verb and noun retrieval in bilingual aphasia and models of language processing. The development of theoretical understandings of language processing are, so far, based mainly on monolingual subjects and these models reflect their word retrieval in one language only. However, there is good reason to assume that when people speak two languages with different underlying forms, verbs and nouns may be affected differently.

The aim of this chapter is an important one given that aphasia in bilinguals and multilinguals is a rather neglected area of research. As a result, there are many significant gaps in the literature regarding issues of assessment and intervention in bilingual aphasia. This is considered a significant omission given that the number of bilingual speakers was acknowledged as outnumbering those of monolingual speakers since the late 1960s.

Specifically, this knowledge base does not reflect the changing demographic picture, in most of the developed world. It is increasingly common for people to speak more than one language due to migration and world globalization. However, despite the recommendations made by peak bodies representing speech pathologists (a term synonymous with speech-language pathologist and speech therapist), which demand equitable services for people from culturally and linguistically diverse backgrounds, the number of bilingual speech pathologists remains low. This means that not only are there insufficient services available for bilingual populations, but also that clinical and theoretical developments in speech pathology have not kept pace with demographic changes. In particular, clinical understanding of language breakdown because of aphasia in two (or more) languages remains poorly understood and clinicians have insufficient knowledge on which to base their interventions.

Chapter II - The role of the right hemisphere for language processing and successful therapeutic interventions in aphasic patients is a matter of debate. New findings indicate a modulation of brain activation in right-hemispheric areas in response to language tasks in chronic non-fluent aphasic patients due to aphasia therapy. These findings show that the therapeutic intervention per se does not change brain activation across all aphasic subjects. However, therapeutic success correlates with a relative decrease of activation in right-hemispheric areas. Most importantly, initial right-hemispheric activation correlates positively with subsequent therapy-induced improvement of language functions. Thus, right-hemispheric activation prior to aphasia therapy strongly predicts therapeutic success. Furthermore, any analysis that is limited to an averaged group of patients seems to be insufficient in order to detect individual and partially opposite brain activation patterns. This chapter discusses the implication of the new findings for the understanding of neural processes involved in the recovery of language functions in aphasic subjects.

Chapter III - Many patients with different degenerative dementias also exhibit aphasia in varying degrees. Recent evidence has suggested that the fluency test might be a powerful assessment to aid in diagnostic decisions of dementia and could be deemed the one-minute mental status examination. Verbal fluency tasks consist of generating words from a semantic category (e.g., animals) or words beginning with a given letter (e.g., the letter 'S') within a specified time limit, such as 60 seconds. The use of the fluency task as a quick mental status exam is not only appealing in its brevity to administer but also in the potential richness of the data acquired. The present chapter presents findings from a study that compared how patients with different degenerative dementia syndromes with aphasia performed on category and letter fluency tasks. Patients with primary progressive aphasia, semantic dementia, and Alzheimer's disease were compared with normal controls on fluency tasks as these three disease conditions are often difficult to distinguish from one another using general cognitive screens and neuroimaging, particularly at the early stages of disease onset. The results from this study comparing these patients with aphasia reveal that category and letter fluency tasks may be more helpful in distinguishing various dementia syndromes from normal controls and from one another than the more general cognitive screens that are typically used to assess dementia. In summary, this chapter expands and improves upon the currently accepted methodology used in the diagnosis of dementia, particularly when aphasia is a core symptom.

Chapter IV - In recent years, the availability of online techniques (i.e., when language comprehension is measured as a sentence unfolds) has given rise to a new line of research complementing traditional findings from offline methodologies and providing finer-grained characterizations of the deficit underlying aphasia. The emerging data question the classic characterization of the agrammatic aphasia comprehension deficit as one of loss of certain structural representations. The present chapter thus provides a review of a slowly but steadily growing body of experimental research into the real-time sentence processing of individuals with agrammatic Broca's aphasia. It draws on evidence that mainly derives from the comprehension of various non-canonical structures (including *wh*-questions, passives, cleft constructions, and NP-movement) as well as pronominal interpretation, and that is based on data from cross-modal lexical decision priming and interference tasks, anomaly detection, word monitoring paradigms, eye tracking and electrophysiology. The chapter discusses the implications of these real-time data for theoretical accounts of the aphasic syndrome and argues for slowed-down processing rather than loss of knowledge representations as the sources of the comprehension deficit.

Chapter V - Dual-route models and right-hemispheric accounts were suggested to predict comprehension of figurative language in healthy speakers as well as in patients with language disorders. In considering cognitive and neural correlates of recent findings, an alternative model of figurative language comprehension will be discussed. The proposed *Linguistic Analysis-Synthesis* (LAS) model states that "synthetic" expressions do not standby to fill in for "analytical" phrases. The LAS model stipulates only gradual differences between analytical and synthetic lexical computations. Recent neuroimaging evidence supports the view that idiomatic phrases are primarily processed within the left inferior frontal gyrus. It is concluded that the use of frequent expressions produced during chitchats is a much more promising technique to treat fluency disorders in aphasia than the use of idiomatic expressions.

Chapter VI – Purpose: To describe clinical characteristics and lateralizing value of postictal perseveration (repetitive verbal behavior) in patients with temporal lobe epilepsy (TLE). Other postictal language disorders (aphasia, paraphasia) are well-described signs in TLE; however, postictal perseveration has not been systematically analyzed so far.

Methods: One hundred and ninety-three videotaped seizures of 55 consecutive patients with refractory TLE and postoperatively seizure-free outcome were analyzed. Postictal perseveration was monitored.

Results: Perseveration was observed during the postictal period in 18 (9%) of the 193 seizures. The phenomenon occurred more frequently after left-sided seizures (16 left-sided and two right-sided; p=0.002). Neither age at epilepsy onset, age at monitoring, duration of epilepsy nor gender were significantly different between patients with and without postictal perseveration.

Chapter VII - Conclusion: Postictal perseveration is a rare phenomenon in TLE but lateralizes the seizure onset zone to the left hemisphere. Our observation can help the presurgical evaluation of TLE because verbal perseveration frequently occurs spontaneously, even in seizures without appropriate postictal language testing.

This chapter will present a general framework for looking at bilingual aphasia and will review issues relevant to the assessment and treatment of anomia in bilingual aphasic adults. Anomia is the most universal symptom in aphasia, and one which patients find frustrating. It is also one of the best studied areas in aphasia, drawing on a large body of knowledge about lexical models, lexical access, and the naming process in non-aphasic adults.

This chapter begins by defining some of the key terminology. The bulk of the chapter is devoted to a discussion of current assessment methods, especially assessment of naming impairments, and a review of studies on the rehabilitation of bilingual aphasia, with a particular focus on the assessment and treatment of naming (or word-finding) The chapter closes with a commentary on various methodological issues and steps to foster more rapid progress in the field of bilingual aphasia.

Chapter VIII - Both structural and functional neuroimaging are rapidly evolving. Neuroimaging has been critical to demonstrating that classic aphasia syndromes arise after stroke because areas of the brain necessary for particular language functions predictably fall in the territory of the same artery. Such syndromes can reflect either permanent damage to the vascular territory or hypoperfusion caused by stenosis or occlusion of the artery. More selective deficits (components of aphasic syndromes) arise when acute damage or hypoperfusion involves only a small part of the vascular territory; or as a result of reorganization after chronic brain damage, such that other components of the aphasia syndrome are assumed by other parts of the brain.

In: Aphasia: Symptoms, Diagnosis and Treatment
Editors: G. Ibanescu, S. Pescariu

ISBN: 978-1-60741-288-5
© 2009 Nova Science Publishers, Inc.

Chapter I

Investigating Grammatical Word Class Distinctions in Bilingual Aphasic Individuals

*Maria Kambanaros**
European University Cyprus, Cyprus

Abstract

This chapter will review two major areas in the aphasiology literature, (i) grammatical word class processing by aphasic individuals and (ii) bilingual aphasia, each of which is essential to an understanding of the topic. The first relates to **grammatical word class processing**, specifically that for **verbs** and **nouns**. This area is extremely important because word-finding difficulties for verbs and nouns are so common in aphasia. Also, the processing differences between verbs and nouns that occur at various levels of linguistic analysis: semantic, syntactic, morphological, and phonological will be highlighted. In addition, an overview of the major research studies that have specifically investigated verb-noun dissociations and the patterns of verb and noun impairments in aphasic syndromes is provided. Evidence from neuroimaging studies is also reviewed. The findings reported will be considered in relation to explanatory models locating the breakdown at either linguistic or neuroanatomical levels.

Furthermore, in this chapter, I will focus on grammatical word class breakdown in the context of bilingual aphasia. This section will highlight what little is known about how verbs and nouns are processed in bilingual patients due to the reliance on monolingual subjects in these studies. I will present up-to-date research available on **investigating grammatical word class distinctions** and, indeed, in different languages, in people with bilingual aphasia.

This focus is also significant for a theoretical understanding of verb and noun retrieval in bilingual aphasia and models of language processing. The development of theoretical understandings of language processing are, so far, based mainly on

---

* Corresponding author: European University Cyprus, Department of Humanities, Program in Speech and Language Therapy, 3 Diogenes, CY-1516 Engomi, Nicosia, Cyprus; E-mail: M.Kambanaros@euc.ac.cy

monolingual subjects and these models reflect their word retrieval in one language only. However, there is good reason to assume that when people speak two languages with different underlying forms, verbs and nouns may be affected differently.

The aim of this chapter is an important one given that aphasia in bilinguals and multilinguals is a rather neglected area of research. As a result, there are many significant gaps in the literature regarding issues of assessment and intervention in bilingual aphasia. This is considered a significant omission given that the number of bilingual speakers was acknowledged as outnumbering those of monolingual speakers since the late 1960s.

Specifically, this knowledge base does not reflect the changing demographic picture, in most of the developed world. It is increasingly common for people to speak more than one language due to migration and world globalization. However, despite the recommendations made by peak bodies representing speech pathologists (a term synonymous with speech-language pathologist and speech therapist), which demand equitable services for people from culturally and linguistically diverse backgrounds, the number of bilingual speech pathologists remains low. This means that not only are there insufficient services available for bilingual populations, but also that clinical and theoretical developments in speech pathology have not kept pace with demographic changes. In particular, clinical understanding of language breakdown because of aphasia in two (or more) languages remains poorly understood and clinicians have insufficient knowledge on which to base their interventions.

Introduction

The aphasiology literature contains many examples of research that address verb retrieval, noun retrieval and word processing. It also includes many published sources that have explored bilingual aphasia. To date, there have been few studies combining the findings of these two areas. As yet, the nature of verb and noun retrieval in bilingual aphasic populations has not been investigated. This chapter provides a literature review of two major areas in aphasiology, grammatical word class processing by aphasic individuals and bilingual aphasia, each of which is essential to an understanding of the topic under exploration. The first relates to potential differences in grammatical word class processing, specifically differences between verb and noun processing. This area is important because word-finding difficulties for verbs and nouns are so common in aphasia. In its simplest definition, aphasia is a disorder of language due to brain damage, most commonly stroke. It often affects language production and comprehension, compromising both spoken and written language. Problems can arise at linguistic levels such as semantics, syntax, morphology and phonology. Aphasia may range from mild to severe, but it almost universally affects the ability to find words, nouns and verbs in particular.

In addition, the findings from studies investigating verb-noun breakdown in aphasia have been so influential in the development of models of language processing. Verbs and nouns can be differentially affected in aphasia (Miceli et al., 1984; Zingeser & Berndt, 1988, 1990), although no consistent patterns have been identified thus far to suggest discrete links between lesion site and verb-noun differences. The review of the literature focuses on the major research studies that have specifically investigated verb-noun dissociations. The findings reported are considered in relation to explanatory models locating the breakdown at either linguistic levels or neuroanatomical differences.

The emphasis on grammatical word class distinctions in this chapter, reflect their common breakdown in aphasia, and the pivotal role of verbs-nouns in communication. This focus is also significant for a theoretical understanding of verb-noun retrieval in bilingual aphasia and models of language processing. The development of theoretical understandings of language processing is so far based mainly on monolingual subjects and these models reflect their word retrieval in one language only. However, there is good reason to assume that when people speak two languages with different underlying forms, verbs and nouns may be affected differently. This issue is important in gaining a deeper understanding of how language is represented for different underlying deep structures.

Moreover, this research is relevant to speech pathology intervention. There is little doubt that cognitive neuropsychological models have been highly influential for aphasia therapy in recent years (Basso & Marangolo, 2000; Bastiaanse, Bosje & Franssen, 1996; Best, Howard, Bruce & Gatehouse, 1997; Best & Nickels, 2000; Drew & Thompson, 1999; Mitchum, Greenwald & Berndt, 2000; Nickels & Best, 1996; Raymer, Thompson, Jacobs & Le Grand, 1993). Once again, most of the models are based on monolingual subjects. Consequently, existing theoretical principles that underpin aphasia therapy planning are restricted to speakers of one language only.

This knowledge base does not reflect the changing demographic picture, in most of the developed world. It is increasingly common for people to speak more than one language due to migration and globalisation. Yet speech pathology, is referred to as a predominantly monolingual or Anglo-dominated profession in an increasing multicultural world (Baker, 2002; Hand, O'Sullivan, Plumer, Gupta, Mackaway et al., 2000; Isaac, 2002; Whitworth & Sjardin, 1993). According to Hand et al., (2000)

> Virtually all the principles and knowledge base upon which the profession operates are of monolingual and monocultural English-speaking culture and language (p. 198).

However, despite the recommendations made by peak bodies representing speech pathologists[1] (American Speech and Hearing Association, 2000; Royal College of Speech and Language Therapists, 1996; Speech Pathology Australia, 1994) which demand equitable services for people from culturally and linguistically diverse backgrounds (CLD), the number of bilingual speech pathologists world-wide remains low (Battle, 1998; Baker, 2002; Cheng, Battle, Murdoch, & Martin, 2001; Roberts, 1998, 2001; Stapleford & Todd, 1998; Whitworth & Sjardin, 1993). This means that not only are there insufficient services available for bilingual populations, but also that clinical and theoretical developments have not kept pace with demographic changes. In particular, clinical understanding of language breakdown because of aphasia in two (or more) languages remains poorly understood and clinicians have insufficient knowledge on which to base their interventions (Kambanaros, 2003; Kambanaros & van Steenbrugge, 2004; Kambanaros, 2009; Kayser, 1998). Furthermore, not only are there

---

[1] Speech Pathologist is synonymous with Speech-Language Pathologist and Speech Therapist.

few bilingual clinicians, there are also few bilingual assessment tools, with only one published bilingual assessment for this population (Paradis & Libben, 1987).

The second part of the literature review discusses language breakdown in the context of bilingual aphasia. This section illustrates what little is known about how verbs and nouns are processed in bilingual patients due to the reliance on monolingual subjects in the majority of studies. Much of the work in the area of verb and noun processing relates to monolingual individuals with aphasia, particularly to speakers of English. Also, comparative aphasiology, the study of aphasia in different languages, is a relatively new area of research. Only in the last decade are the communication difficulties (including verb-noun breakdown) in aphasic patients from different linguistic and cultural backgrounds documented in the international English aphasiology or 'mainstream' literature (Roberts, 2001). Moreover, aphasia in bilinguals is a rather neglected area of research. As a result, there are many significant gaps in the literature regarding issues of assessment and intervention in bilingual aphasia. This is considered a significant omission given that the number of bilingual speakers was acknowledged as outnumbering those of monolingual speakers since the late sixties (Mackey, 1967).

One reason for the lack of research in this area relates to the substantial methodological difficulties facing researchers (Ardila, 1998; Grosjean, 1998). These difficulties sometimes relate to subject selection criteria and assessment measures (Chary, 1986; Grosjean, 1998; Roberts, 1998). A further difficulty is related to understanding how languages are stored in the brain. Studies investigating the localization of two languages in the bilingual brain have focused on identifying the similarities and/or differences in the cortical areas associated with acquiring these languages. Functional neuroimaging research postulates that language is lateralized and organized similarly in the brain for bilingual and monolingual speakers (Klein, Zattore, Milner, Meyer & Evans, 1994). Paradis (2008) has suggested that the cerebral organization underlying communication abilities is specific to language in general rather than to one language in particular, that is, the two language systems of bilingual speakers are likely to utilize the same or adjacent neural structures in the brain. On the other hand, clinical studies of bilingual aphasia have provided some evidence that a bilingual speaker may selectively lose one language and sparing the other, suggesting that the neural representation of the two languages is differentially organised (Albert & Obler, 1978; Fabbro, 1999; Kehayia, Singer & Jarema, 1996; Paradis, 1983).

This focus on cross-linguistic issues is also important for two additional reasons. Firstly, the assessment of aphasia in both languages is likely to increase diagnostic accuracy and provide a comprehensive picture of residual communication ability for use in planning treatment. This is reinforced by Paradis (2001) who states:

> …it is important for one to be aware of the particular manifestations of aphasic symptoms in a given language or family of languages, namely, to avoid misdiagnosis (p.5).

He further acknowledged that the same underlying lesion may cause differing surface manifestations in different languages, and that one must interpret the patients' pattern in terms of its significance for each language. Secondly, treatment of - and service delivery to -

clients afflicted by aphasia should be a key issue for clinicians. Speech pathologists devote considerable time to the treatment of word retrieval deficits and to identifying useful therapy techniques and models of service delivery best suited for each client according to their level of breakdown. To date, no clear, predictable relationship has emerged between the kind of word-finding problem such as semantic errors, and the most appropriate treatment in aphasia (Best & Nickels, 2000). By inference, much remains unknown about treating word production breakdowns in bilingual aphasia (Conroy, Sage, & Lambon Ralph, 2006).

Bilingual individuals can acquire a second language early or later in life. This language can be learnt formally, through schooling, or informally in communicative situations. The two languages are often used for different purposes in diverse domains of life and with different people. This has led to the misconception that bilingual speakers have equal and faultless fluency in each of their languages, what has been called "the two monolinguals in one person viewpoint" (Grosjean, 1989). However, it is a fact that bilinguals rarely have equal abilities in their two languages (Grosjean, 1989, 1997; Kohnert, Hernandez & Bates, 1998). Bilingual individuals can show different levels of proficiency in the different linguistic components of a language (e.g. lexical semantics, morphology, syntax, phonology) as well as in the different language modalities (e.g. auditory/written comprehension, spoken/written language).

Grammatical Word Class Processing

The issue of how people with aphasia access and/or retrieve verbs and nouns is extremely complex and there are many different views put forward in the literature as to the breakdown of the processes involved. The finding by many researchers that verb retrieval is more difficult than noun retrieval in aphasia (Berndt et al., 1997; Caramazza & Hillis, 1991; Jonkers & Bastiaanse, 1998; Kambanaros, 2008; Miceli et al., 1984; Orpwood & Warrington, 1995; Rapp & Caramazza, 1998; Tranel et al., 2001; Tsapkini et al., 2002; Zingeser & Berndt, 1990) is only one of several findings. The different nature of verb-noun dissociations in aphasia is possibly because of the variability in verb/noun meanings; the complex relationship between verbs and nouns (e.g., instrumentality, name-relation); the different patterns of verb-noun dissociations and the different aphasia syndromes; the differing linguistic and neurophysiological explanations for the levels of breakdown; methodological issues; and the differential structures between languages. Each of these issues will be addressed below.

Verb and Noun Variability

Verbs and nouns are highly variable in meaning. Verbs denote events i.e. what happens to things, including actions, while nouns typically denote entities such as people, animals and objects. Due to their individual characteristics, verbs and nouns may be represented and processed differently (Damasio & Tranel, 1993; Gainotti et al., 1995). It is assumed that verb knowledge is subserved by regions important for knowledge associated with actions such as the frontal cortex near motor/premotor areas, whereas knowledge about nouns is supposedly localized in brain regions that also subserve the processing of more general semantic knowledge about concrete properties of objects like the inferior temporal lobe.

Furthermore, a verb's central meaning (e.g. "*to write*," is different from "*to read*") is linked to two kinds of information: thematic role assignment and argument structure. In simple terms, the verb's central meaning determines the "*who does what to whom*". More specifically, argument structure refers to the number and types of arguments the verb requires. For example, the central meaning of the verb "*to swim*" determines that it has only one argument, the verb "*to throw*" has two arguments, an agent and a patient; and the verb "*to sell*" has three arguments, agent, theme and recipient. A thematic role is assigned to each argument in the form of noun phrases that provide additional meaning allowing the verb to stand within a particular sentence e.g. the noun phrase "*the donkey*" has a different thematic role (sentential meaning) in "*the donkey carries the man*" than in "*the man carries the donkey*". Moreover, sentences must satisfy the complement structure of a verb and be grammatically correct in relation to the Projection Principle (Chomsky, 1981), that is, all arguments must be specified in order for the sentence to be acceptable to the listener.

The many attempts to unravel the processes underlying verb-noun differences have relied on words that can be pictured. For example, nouns have been represented by pictures of concrete objects (e.g. car) and verbs picturable actions (e.g. driving). Some subjects with aphasia have shown a selective difficulty naming pictures of actions in comparison to pictures of objects and vice-versa (Berndt, Haendiges et al., 1997; Berndt, Mitchum et al., 1997; Damasio & Tranel, 1993; Daniele et al., 1994; McCarthy & Warrington, 1985; Silveri & Di Betta, 1997). For some of these patients the deficit was identified at the conceptual level (Daniele et al., 1994; McCarthy & Warrington, 1985; Silveri & Di Betta, 1997) rather than one of lexical retrieval.

Other investigators have argued that picture-naming tasks favour the production of nouns (Kohn et al., 1989; Williams & Canter, 1987) because they represent concrete objects that are easily pictured. In contrast, subjects with verb impairments may have difficulty identifying the action component when naming static pictures and may fail to name actions for that reason (Berndt et al., 1997).[2] Similarly, verb deficits for some patients appeared to camouflage a more general semantic deficit for action names rather than a grammatical class "verb" deficit (Daniele et al., 1994; McCarthy & Warrington, 1985). It is conceivable then that verb-noun differences in some subjects could be linked to semantic differences between the word classes at the level of the central semantic system that is, a category specific deficit for action/object words. This has lead to the proposal that the observed dissociations reflect the organization of semantic knowledge rather than effects of the grammatical properties of words (Breedin et al., 1998, Marshall et al., 1996; McCarthy & Warrington, 1985).

An additional factor impacting on the semantic differences between action and object names is *imageability*. Action pictures are rated as less *imageable* (have fewer semantic features) than object pictures (Bird, Howard & Franklin, 2000; Luzzatti et al., 2002). Yet, imageability is not often controlled for in picture-naming studies because pictured stimuli are

---

[2] However verb-noun dissociations were also found when video taped stimuli of actions and objects were used instead of pictures (Berndt, Mitchum et al., 1997).

considered highly imageable (Jonkers, 1998; Jonkers & Bastiaanse, 1996; Nickels, 1995). However it has been argued that not all pictured stimuli are equally imageable (Bird et al., 2000) especially with respect to verbs. Not much was known about the effect of imageability on verb retrieval until the studies by Bird et al., 2000; Luzzatti et al., 2002, reported better noun than verb retrieval in some individual subjects because of their higher imageability. However, the account that verb-noun differences arise not because of real grammatical word class differences, but rather because of imageability differences, and specifically that there are no differences between verbs and nouns if imageability is controlled for (Bird et al., 2000; Luzzatti et al., 2002; Marshall, Chiat, Robson & Pring, 1995/6) has not gone unchallenged (Berndt, Haendiges, Burton, & Mitchum, 2002; Caramazza & Shapiro, 2002).

Moreover, other findings have suggested that imageability differences are not limited to verbs compared to concrete nouns, as suggested by Bird et al., (2000) but that words within each grammatical category can show an effect of imageability. This means that in the verb category there are action words that are considered more imageable than others and the same applies to nouns. For example, Kemmerer and Tranel (2000) using ratings from normative data (Fiez & Tranel 1997) reported that brain-injured subjects found highly imageable verbs (e.g. stirring) easier to retrieve than low imageable verbs (e.g. sticking). Similarly, nouns rated lower in imageability are less well retrieved in aphasia than nouns of higher imageability (Franklin, Howard & Patterson, 1995; Nickels, 1995; Nickels & Howard, 1995).

In addition, the difference between action and object names has been linked to the loss of functional and perceptual knowledge respectively (Bird et al., 2000; Marshall, Chiat, et al., 1996; Marshall, Pring, Chiat & Robson, 1996). Bird et al., (2000) claimed that verbs, compared to nouns, have more functional than perceptual attributes and that functional feature damage will result in impaired verb naming. Furthermore, within the category of nouns, non-living objects or artifacts are represented by more functional information (what one does with them) than living nouns. Thus, Bird and colleagues (2000) hypothesized that damage to areas of the brain where primarily functional features are encoded may adversely affect both verb and inanimate noun retrieval. On the other hand, perceptual feature impairment would result in spared verb naming but impaired retrieval of animate nouns.

The conclusion by Bird and colleagues (2000), in which they reduced verb-noun differences to loss of either functional or perceptual feature representations, has been seriously criticized in the literature (Berndt et al., 2002; Druks, 2002; Shapiro & Caramazza, 2001). Generally, these assumptions fail to account for the numerous cases of subjects with selective verb-noun deficits that defy explanations under a functional–perceptual or imageability account.

Despite the complexity and contradictory findings in the literature related to grammatical word class processing, a robust finding is that grammatical class effects may arise in subjects with aphasia. According to Luzzatti and colleagues (2002):

"verb-noun dissociations cannot be simply discarded as an artifact resulting from unbalanced word frequency or imageability, but have to be accepted as a genuine part-of-speech effect" (p. 442).

The Complex Relationship between Verbs and Nouns

There is also growing evidence that verbs and nouns belonging to different semantic categories respectively are affected by aphasia. With regards to verb processing, studies targeting specific verb types are few, possibly because of difficulties in devising suitable stimulus materials (Fietz & Tranel, 1997). However, findings from studies investigating verbs from different lexical-semantic categories have revealed that the verb's central meaning can be selectively impaired while knowledge of argument structure and subcategorization frames is preserved (Breedin & Martin, 1996; Marshall et al., 1996). For example, the subject described by Marshall and colleagues, (RG), found it more difficult to access information about the type of event encoded by the verb (e.g. skate versus slide) but had little difficult assigning thematic roles to the verb. This disruption is intriguing because verb deficits are typically assumed to result from the different grammatical role verbs play in a sentence relative to nouns.

Furthermore, research in the last two decades (Bastiaanse, 1991; Bastiaanse & Jonkers, 1998; Breedin, Boronat, Saffran & Shipley, 1999; Breedin & Martin, 1996; Breedin, Saffran & Schwartz, 1998; Druks & Shallice, 2000; Jonkers, 1998; Jonkers & Bastiaanse, 1996; 2007; Kemmerer & Tranel, 2000) has shown that the retrieval of a specific semantic/conceptual category of verbs, namely instrumental verbs, can be compromised by aphasia. Instrumental verbs are verbs referring to actions that require a man-made instrument. For example, the verb *"sweep"* necessitates a broom. *"Climb"* however is not instrumental. For instrumental verbs, the instrument information (e.g., broom) is integral to their meaning (Jackendoff, 1990; Nagy & Gentner, 1990) and the presence of this instrument gives the verb a more specific meaning in relation to other verbs e.g., *sweep* versus *clean*.

Some aphasic subjects found retrieving verbs for actions that involve an instrument more difficult than those for actions that do not (Berndt & Haendiges, 2000; Breedin & Martin, 1996; Kemmerer & Tranel, 2000). However, the opposite has been reported in anomic subjects, that is instrumental verbs are easier to retrieve than other verbs (Jonkers, 1998; Jonkers & Bastiaanse, 1996, 1998, 2007). It has been postulated (Breedin et al., 1998) that verb retrieval for some aphasic individuals is facilitated by (additional) semantic/conceptual complexity at the level of the (verb) lemma.

Moreover, one additional factor found to affect instrumental verb retrieval in aphasia is name relation. Name relation refers to noun-verb pairs such as *"hammer"* and *"to hammer"* where the one (phonological) word form represents a noun as well as a verb. Recent studies suggest that name relation can have a positive, facilitating effect on instrumental verb retrieval in some aphasic subjects with selective verb impairments (Breedin et al., 1999; Jonkers & Bastiaanse, 1996; Kremin, 1994; Kemmerer & Tranel, 2000). This has particularly been the case for anomic aphasic individuals with good comprehension for verbs and nouns (Jonkers & Bastiaanse, 1996; Kremin, 1994). The positive effect of name relation on instrumental verb retrieval in anomia is claimed to operate at the phonological form/lexeme level because of the phonological relationship between the noun and verb forms (Bastiaanse, 1991; Jonkers, 1998).

In contrast, a large number of studies have investigated the retrieval of different semantic categories of nouns in aphasia. For example, there is extensive research showing that brain injury may produce the selective disruption of knowledge about living things or animate objects (Caramazza & Shelton, 1998; Hart, Berndt & Caramazza, 1985; Hillis & Caramazza, 1991; Tranel, Damasio & Damasio, 1997; Warrington & Shallice, 1984). Though less common, knowledge about man-made artifacts or inanimate nouns (Hillis & Caramazza, 1991; Damasio, 1990; Ferreira, Giusiano, & Poncet, 1997; Sacchett & Humphries, 1992; Warrington &McCarthy, 1983) can be selectively disrupted by brain injury.

In some studies the deficits have involved more specific semantic categories within these broad categories e.g. animals (Hart & Gordon, 1992), fruits and vegetables (Farah & Wallace, 1992; Hart, Berndt & Caramazza, 1985) or tools (Damasio, Gabowski, Tranel, Hichwa & Damasio, 1996; Tranel, Damasio & Damasio, 1997). The fact that specific semantic categories of nouns can be selectively damaged or spared after brain injury is interpreted as evidence for either the separate neural representation of categories such as animals, tools etc., or for specialized neural processing networks relaying semantic information related to each category. For example, when retrieving the names of different animals particular features such as colour, shape, size etc. (Saffran & Schwartz, 1994; Warrington & Shallice, 1984) may be impaired rather than the category per se.

Similarly, studies have revealed that some aphasic subjects have more difficulties retrieving instrumental nouns denoting manipulable instruments including tools, with a relative preservation of the ability to name other common nouns/objects (Buxbaum & Saffran, 1998; Damasio et al., 1996; Laiacona & Capitani, 2001). Knowledge about different types of nouns/objects is linked to the different memory systems. The processing of instrumental nouns such as tools (e.g., hammer, saw) has been linked to procedural memory subserved by the left frontal/basal ganglia circuitry (Ullman et al., 1997) while non-manipulated nouns/objects are part of declarative (explicit) memory subserved by left temporal cortical areas. However, studies that have investigated for the effects of instrumentality on verb retrieval in anomia have not done so for noun retrieval.

Verb-noun Dissociations and Aphasia Type

A contradictory pattern of verb-noun breakdown has been described in relation to different types of aphasia. To date, five separate patterns of performance have been identified. These include:

1. Impaired verb retrieval with agrammatic/Broca's aphasia
2. Impaired noun retrieval with Wernicke's/anomic aphasia
3. Impaired verb retrieval for all subjects with aphasia
4. Impaired verb retrieval with Wernicke's/anomic aphasia
5. No differential impairment for verbs and nouns in aphasia

Goodglass, Klein, Carey, and Jones (1966) were the first to report differential noun and verb performance in English monolingual brain-injured patients using picture naming. They found that subjects with Brocas' aphasia were mainly impaired in naming action verbs and subjects with anomia showed a prevalent impairment in naming object nouns. Their seminal study provided the impetus for later neurolinguistic studies seeking to confirm this double dissociation for grammatical class words (verbs and nouns) in Broca's aphasia (Goodglass, 1993; Marin, Saffran & Schwartz, 1976; Myerson & Goodglass, 1972) and anomia (Zingeser & Berndt, 1988).

For close to four decades, researchers have continued to investigate verb-noun dissociations in aphasia using picture naming. Their findings reinforce earlier claims that selective verb impairments are mainly found in nonfluent, agrammatic patients with an anterior cortical lesion that includes Broca's area (Berndt et al., 1997; Breedin et al., 1998; Breen & Warrington, 1994; Kim & Thompson, 2000; Manning & Warrington, 1996; McCarthy & Warrington, 1985; Marshall, Pring & Chiat, 1998; Shapiro et al., 2000; Zingeser & Berndt, 1990).

Interestingly, this finding holds true for languages other than English such as Chinese (Bates, Chen, Tzeng, Li & Opie, 1991), Danish (Jensen, 2000), Dutch (Bastiaanse, 1991; Jonkers, 1998; Jonkers & Bastiaanse, 1996), Finnish (Laine, Kujala, Niemi, & Uusipaikka, 1992), German (De Blesser & Kauschke, 2002), Hungarian (Osman-Sagi, 1987), Italian (Daniele, Guistolisi, Silveri, Colosimo & Gainotti, 1994; Luzzati, Raggi, Zonco, Pistarini, Contardi et al., 2002; Miceli, Silveri, Villa & Caramazza, 1984; Miceli, Silveri, Noncentini & Caramazza, 1988; Silveri & Di Betta, 1997) and Greek (Tsapkini, Jarema & Kehayia, 2002).

Researchers have also found the opposite pattern for aphasia patients with posterior lesions of the left hemisphere, that of, impaired noun retrieval with relatively spared verb naming. Again this has been demonstrated in a number of languages: English (Berndt et al., 1997; Berndt, Haendiges & Wozniak, 1997; Breen & Warrington, 1994; Caramazza & Hillis, 1991; Shapiro, Shelton & Caramazza, 2000; Zingeser & Berndt, 1990), Chinese (Bates, Chen, Tzeng, Li & Opie, 1991; Chen & Bates, 1998), French (Bachoud-Levi & Dupoux, 2003), Italian (Daniele et al., 1994; Luzzatti et al., 2002; Miceli et al., 1984; Miozzo, et al., 1994) and Hungarian (Osman-Sagi, 1987).

There have also been recent reports of selective verb deficits in aphasic subjects with posterior lesions/fluent aphasia in languages such as: Dutch (Bastiaanse & Jonkers, 1998; Jonkers, 1998; Jonkers & Bastiaanse, 1996), English (Berndt & Haendiges, 2000; Berndt et al., 1997; McCann & Edwards, 2002), German (De Blesser & Kauschke, 2002), Italian (Luzzatti et al., 2002), and Greek (Kambanaros, 2008; Tsapkini et al., 2002).

Contrary to the above findings a number of other studies have demonstrated greater difficulty with verb processing compared to noun processing for all aphasic subjects regardless of lesion site (anterior or posterior). This has been reported in English (Berndt, et al., 1997; Caramazza & Hillis, 1991; Daniele et al., 1994; Hillis & Caramazza, 1995; Kohn, Lorch & Pearson, 1989; Manning & Warrington, 1996; Marshall et al, 1998; McCarthy & Warrington, 1985; Williams & Canter, 1987), Dutch (Bastiaanse & Jonkers, 1998; Jonkers & Bastiaanse, 1996), French (Kremin, 1994) and Italian (Basso, Razzano, Faglioni, Zanobio, 1990).

Of particular importance is the observation that the majority of aphasic subjects with noun/verb retrieval impairments do not show the same difficulty in comprehension. However, there are exceptions (Daniele et al., 1994; McCarthy & Warrington, 1985; Miceli et al., 1988; Silveri & Di Betta, 1997 Shapiro et al., 2000).

Thus far, the review suggests a highly complex and apparently contradictory picture. This complexity could be partly explained by poor test constructions and subject selection criteria (Bastiaanse & Jonkers, 1998). For example, not all studies had controlled for variables that affect verb and noun retrieval. In addition, not all studies defined their specific subject group. For example studies involving subjects with fluent aphasia could have included subjects with different aphasia syndromes such as Wernicke's, anomic and conduction aphasia, a factor that could have influenced the results.

A potential reason for the contradictory findings relates to the fact that explanations for this dissociation tend to fall into two main camps, neurophysiological explanations (Damasio & Tranel, 1993; Miozzo et al., 1994) and psycholinguistic explanations (Bastiaanse, 1991; Berndt & Haendiges, 2000; Caramazza & Hillis, 1991; Miceli et al., 1984; Zingeser & Berndt, 1990). In the next section these two possible explanations alluded to above are described in detail.

Differing Psycholinguistic and Neurophysiological Explanations for Levels of Breakdown

Neurophysiological explanation

Several researchers have attributed verb-noun dissociations to different cortical lesions in the left hemisphere (Daniele et al., 1994; Ferreira et al., 1997; Glosser & Donofrio, 2001; Luzzatti et al., 2002; Miozzo et al., 1994; Tranel et al., 2001). Lesion studies have fostered the assumption that verb and noun retrieval may each be mediated by different neural networks, with more involvement of the left posterior frontal cortex, including motor-processing regions, in the retrieval of action words and more involvement of the left temporal cortex, including visual object-processing regions, in the retrieval of object names (Caramazza & Hillis, 1991; Damasio & Tranel, 1993; Miozzo et al., 1994; Manning & Warrington, 1996; Pulvermuller, 1999).

Additional evidence supporting the differential processing of nouns and verbs can also be found in imaging studies, using Positron Emission Tomography (PET), functional Magnetic Resonance Imaging (fMRI), Event Related Potentials (ERP), repetitive Transcranial Magnetic Stimulation (rTMS) and electrophysiological approaches in healthy, non brain-injured individuals. Some PET studies have revealed separate activation patterns for verbs compared to nouns (Martin, Haxby, Lalonde, Wiggs & Ungerleider, 1995; Perani, Cappa, Schnur, Tettamanti, Collina et al., 1999; Tranel, Damasio & Damasio, 1997). Other studies confirm electrocortical differences between noun and verbs over widespread cortical areas, specifically, that action verbs elicited activity above the premotor, motor and prefrontal cortices and nouns over the temporo-occipital cortices (Pulvermüller, Preissl, Lutzenberger & Birbaumer, 1996; Pulvermuller, Lutzenberger & Preissl, 1999; Pulvermuller, Harle, & Friedhelm 2001).

Unfortunately, some of the above studies that attribute naming of actions and objects to different brain regions reported conflicting results in regards to postulated activation sites for action naming. For example, in a recent rTMS study, Shapiro, Pascual-Leone, Mottaghy,

Gangitano & Caramazza, (2001) found that action naming was exclusively dependent on frontal regions, however in the PET study by Martin et al., (1995) activation of the left middle temporal gyrus, rather than the left prefrontal cortex, occurred during generation of action words. Also, verb activation patterns using PET were found in both anterior and posterior regions including Broca's and Wernicke's areas and the pre-motor cortex (Hadar, Palti & Hendler, 2002). In addition, fMRI findings have failed to support prefrontal or parietal activation for action words (Kable, Lease-Spellmeyer & Chatterjee, 2002). Similarly, other PET studies have identified cortical areas common to both object and action naming in normal subjects (Tyler, Russell, Fadili & Moss, 2001; Warburton, Wise, Price, Weiller, Hadar et al., 1996). This finding is supported by recent imaging work in a large group of stroke patients specifically identifying the superior temporal gyrus including Wernicke's area as crucial for naming and understanding both object and action words (Hillis, Tuffiash, Wityk & Barker, 2002).

Recently, in a study using lesion reconstruction methods based on MRI and CT brain imaging in a sample of 20 monolingual Italian aphasic patients, noun impairments were found to involve lesions in the medial part of the middle and left temporal gyri while verb impairments revealed either the left posterior temporal lobe and inferior parietal lesions, or extensive left fronto-temporal involvement (Aggujaro, Crepaldi, Pistarini, Taricco & Luzzatti, 2006).

Furthermore, studies investigating verb-noun dissociations in aphasia have included verb-impaired subjects with "atypical" lesions. Interestingly, there are several reports of patients with verb processing deficits not involving the left frontal regions but more posterior temporo-parietal areas (Luzzatti, et al., 2002) and subcortical structure involvement (Jonkers & Bastiaanse, 1996; Luzzatti et al., 2002; Tsapkini et al., 2002).

Of interest is the finding that the evidence from neuropsychological studies suggesting different neural substrates for verbs and nouns is not entirely supported by neuroimaging research. It is possible that knowledge about actions and objects is represented within a non-differentiated distributed system over a widespread cortical network (Hadar et al., 2002; Tyler et al., 2001; Pulvermuller et al., 1999).

Psycholinguistic explanation

Theoretical models of normal lexical access in production have been applied to the findings to specifically explain verb/action and/or noun/object (word) retrieval deficits during picture naming in (monolingual) aphasia. One very influential model of word production is Levelt's (1989) *blueprint for the speaker*. In this model, the speech production process comprises of four stages: *message generation*, *grammatical encoding*, *phonological encoding*, and *articulation*. Each stage in the model has its own autonomous processing component: *the conceptualizer*, *the formulator* and *the articulator* respectively.

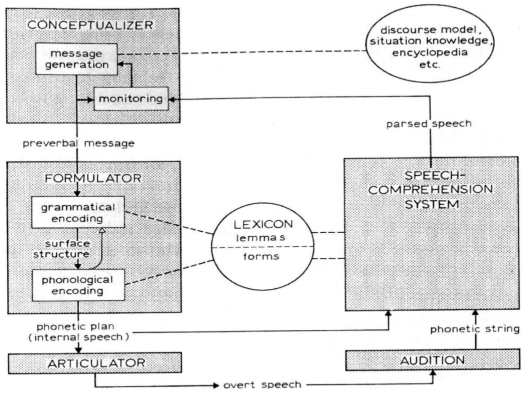

Figure 1. Levelt's blueprint for the speaker
(Levelt, 1989, *Speaking*, p. 9)

In this modular system, each component operates independently and there is no interaction or cascading of activation between the components (hence the modularity principle). Each of the three processing components contains a number of procedures that make up the speaker's procedural knowledge. The procedures operate on the declarative (or factual) knowledge that is stored in the speaker's mental lexicon.

This model (and others) relies on breaking word retrieval into two discrete stages:

a) *lemma selection* and b) *lexeme retrieval* to make the process clear (Dell, 1986; Goodglass, 1993; Levelt, 1989; Levelt, Roelofs & Meyer, 1999).

The lemma is an abstract, language-specific form of the intended word. At the level of the lemma, semantic - and syntactic properties of the word including attachable inflections are specified but not its phonological form (Levelt, 1989). Lemma retrieval is conceptually driven (Levelt, 1989; Levelt, Schriefers, Vorberg, Meyer, Pechmann & Havinga, 1991; Levelt, Roelofs & Meyer, 1999; Roelofs, 2000). For example, during picture naming a speaker must name the pictured object/action (e.g., say "*hammer*" when presented with a pictured hammer). The information in the picture (e.g. the noun-hammer) is termed a *message concept* needing verbalization (Levelt et al., 1999). The preverbal message is received by the *formulator*, and 'translated' by the *grammatical encoder*, (a subcomponent of the formulator) as proposed by Levelt (1989). For grammatical encoding the semantic and syntactic information (i.e. the lemma information) of a lexical entry is needed. In the case of an object name (e.g. hammer), a *noun lemma* is activated which specifies other grammatical information about the noun, such as plurality and grammatical gender. At the second stage of word retrieval, the lexeme or word form corresponding to the selected lemma is phonologically specified. Lexemes contain information about the phonology (number of syllables, prosody, segmentation) and morphology (verb/noun inflections) of a word (Levelt, 1989; Levelt et al., 1999).

Evidence in favour of deficits at both levels of lexical access has been provided. Overall the verb deficit in non-fluent/agrammatic subjects is attributed to a breakdown at the level of the lemma (Bastiaanse, 1991; Jonkers, 1998) whereas in subjects with anomia it is assumed either at the level of the phonological word form (Caramazza & Hillis, 1991; Jonkers, 1998) or at the lemma level (Berndt, Mitchum et al., 1997; Berndt, Haendiges et al., 1997; Berndt et al., 2002).

Specifically in this section, a detailed linguistic explanation focusing on naming breakdown at either the level of lexical – semantics, lemma or at the word-form level will be discussed. Four accounts have been postulated to explain the dissociations between verbs and nouns in aphasia. These are: the semantic-conceptual account; the syntactic account; the morphological account and the lexical account (Chen & Bates, 1998).

Semantic-conceptual account: A large number of researchers attribute grammatical class deficits to a breakdown at the level of lexical-semantics. Their findings suggest that selective verb-noun retrieval impairments occur as a result of a disruption in accessing the central meaning associated with either the verb or noun prior to production, that is, at the level of the lemma (Bates et al., 1991; Bates et al., 1998; Breedin et al., 1998; Druks & Shallice, 2000; Ferreira et al., 1997a; Ferreira et al, 1997b; Gainotti et al., 1995; Kim & Thompson, 2000; Luzzatti et al., 2002; Magnie et al., 1999; Marshall et al., 1996; McCarthy & Warrington, 1985; Moss et al., 1998; Shelton, Fouch & Caramazza, 1998; Silveri & Di Betta, 1997; Williams & Canter, 1987; Zingeser & Berndt, 1990). However for many subjects in the above studies comprehension for verbs and nouns remains largely intact.

Syntactic account: This account attributes verb-noun dissociations to the greater syntactic complexity of verbs compared to nouns because of their pivotal role in sentence construction. Evidence in support of the syntactic account is based on earlier reported correlations between verb deficits and impaired sentence production typically observed in many patients with agrammatic speech (Miceli et al., 1984, 1989; Myerson & Goodglass, 1972; Saffran, 1982; Saffran, Schwartz & Marin, 1980). Similarly, studies on agrammatism have identified specific syntactic properties of verbs that deter verb retrieval in agrammatic speakers such as the presence of increasing argument structure (Kim & Thompson, 2000; Kiss, 2000; Thompson et al., 1997) and the transitivity/intransitivity of the verb (Bastiaanse & Jonkers, 1998; Caplan & Hanna, 1998; Jonkers, 1998; Luzzatti et al., 2002).

In contrast, to the above, findings from recent studies have revealed that firstly, verb deficits are not always associated with impaired sentence production in agrammatism (Bastiaanse & Jonkers, 1998) and secondly, subjects with fluent aphasia also show impaired verb retrieval (Bastiaanse, 1991; Berndt et al., 1997; Breedin & Martin, 1996; Jonkers, 1998; Luzzatti et al., 2002). Furthermore, the syntactic account is implausible because it cannot account for double dissociations (where nouns are more impaired than verbs) and for selective verb impairments in aphasia without agrammatism.

Morphological account: This account hinges on the suggestion that verbs are more difficult to produce than nouns for agrammatic speakers because of their greater morphological complexity related to tense and agreement marking (Caramazza & Berndt, 1985). However this account can be rejected for two main reasons. First, specific morphological difficulties have been recently described for nouns in the light of intact verb inflections (Shapiro, Shelton & Caramazza, 2000). Second, verb/noun dissociations occur even in uninflected languages with no grammatical morphology (Bates et al., 1991) and in languages with comparable morphological distinctions between nouns and verbs (Osman-Sagi, 1987; Tsapkini et al., 2001; 2002). For example, Tsapkini and colleagues (2002) present the case of a monolingual Greek-speaking non-fluent aphasic patient who had difficulties producing inflected verb forms though he was able to perform equally complex morphological operations with nouns.

Lexical account: This account assumes that verb-noun dissociations are the result of a breakdown at the level of the word's form or lexeme, rather than at the lemma. The impairment is located at the level of phonological processing or as a deficit in the phonological output lexicon that is organized according to grammatical category (Breen & Warrington, 1994; Caramazza & Hillis, 1991; Hillis & Caramazza, 1995; Kay & Ellis, 1987; Manning & Warrington, 1996; Marshall et al., 1998; Miceli et al., 1988; Tsapkini et al., 2002). This conclusion is often obtained in the absence of major syntactic and semantic deficits.

It is proposed that verbs and nouns are stored in independent subsystems, possibly with distinct neural substrates and pathways for retrieving the phonological (or orthographic) form (Caramazza & Hillis, 1991; Manning & Warrington, 1996; Miceli et al., 1988; Miozzzo, Soardi & Cappa, 1994)[3]. Therefore, impaired access to either subsystem or pathways might disrupt the production of verbs/nouns and result in form-specific problems in one modality (e.g. writing) but not another (e.g. naming).

Methodological Issues

Researchers have employed a wide range of methodological approaches to investigate verb versus noun retrieval, and the research findings are difficult to compare because of the different methodologies used. The range of approaches is summarized in Table 1.

An additional methodological issue making verb/noun retrieval research complex relates to the different ways subjects with aphasia have been asked to respond to the verb/noun stimuli during testing (see Table 1). For example, several researchers have noted differing patterns in the retrieval of verbs or nouns depending on the retrieval context, that is, retrieval in *single word* versus *sentences*. For example, Manning and Warrington (1996) described a subject who was able to name objects in a picture-naming task but was unable to name the same objects in a sentence completion task. The reverse has also been reported, that is, a subject who was poor at naming single objects showed improved object naming when he was asked to produce object names using a sentence completion task (Zingeser & Berndt, 1988). In contrast, Jonkers and Bastiaanse (1998) described two subjects with a selective disorder for verbs at the single word level but no such deficit in connected speech. This finding is different from what is typically described in the literature, namely impaired verb retrieval typically associated with poor sentence processing and preserved verb retrieval with spared sentence processing (Zingeser & Berndt, 1990). The range of elicitation techniques used in research investigating noun and verb retrieval in (monolingual) aphasia is reported in Table 1.

In addition, findings from recent single subject studies revealed that difficulties retrieving verbs or nouns may be related to a specific modality of output. One subject (Druks & Shallice, 2000) was very poor at naming verbs (and nouns) presented as pictures but came close to maximum performance naming the same verbs when the actions were acted out in front of him or when he was asked to mime the action or his body was manipulated in order for him to name the verb. Furthermore, others have reported subjects with selective impairments in oral versus written production of single verbs (Caramazza & Hillis, 1991) and vice-versa in both single-word and sentence production tasks (Rapp & Caramazza, 1998) or only for written sentences (Berndt & Haendiges, 2000). Most striking is the report of a double dissociation of grammatical category by modality, that is, greater difficulties when orally producing nouns than verbs and greater difficulties in writing verbs than nouns at both single word and sentence levels (Rapp & Caramazza, 2002). However, it should be noted that modality-specific grammatical word class effects have not always been found in studies investigating verb/noun retrieval deficits across a wide range of tasks (Miozzo et al., 1994; Silveri & Di Betta, 1997).

Despite the different elicitation techniques the vast majority of studies have used picture naming to investigate verb and noun retrieval in aphasia, because picture naming offers certain advantages over other methods (Goodglass, 1993; Kohn et al., 1989). Subjects with aphasia usually understand this task and are often already familiar with it because of its common usage in clinical assessment and therapy. Pictures are easily standardized and usually elicit one response/target, and allow researchers to interpret unintelligible responses (because they can also see the target). In addition, individuals with aphasia do not typically have agnosia and so cope well with picture recognition tasks (Goodglass, 1993; Kohn & Goodglass, 1985; Nickels, 1995). Nevertheless, picture naming is obviously restricted by the fact that abstract nouns and verbs are difficult to visualize and portray in picture format. For example, a picture of "*faith*" or "*believing*" is more difficult to portray than "*car*" and "*driving*".

Others suggest that nouns and verbs are organised in a single semantic system (Moss, Davies, Jeppeson, McLellan & Tyler, 1998).

Table 1. The range of elicitation techniques used in research investigating noun and verb retrieval in aphasia.

Elicitation technique	Researchers
Naming to definition	Berndt, Mitchum, Haendiges, & Sandson, 1997; Druks & Shallice, 2000; Marshall, Pring & Chiat, 1998; Marshall, Pring, Chiat & Robson, 1995/6; Zingeser & Berndt, 1990
Sentence completion/construction	Bastiaanse, 1991; Berndt & Haendiges, 2000; Berndt, Haendiges, Mitchum, Sandson, 1997; Berndt, Mitchum, Haendiges, & Sandson, 1997; Berndt, Haendiges, & Wozniak, 1997; Breedin & Martin, 1996; Breedin et al., 1998; Jensen, 2000; Kohn, Lorch & Pearson, 1989; Manning & Warrington, 1996; Marshall et al., 1998; McCall, Cox, Shelton, Weinrich, 1997; Thompson, Lange, Schneider & Shapiro, 1997;
Naming from a video-taped scene	Berndt, Mitchum, Haendiges, & Sandson, 1997; Berndt, Haendiges, & Wozniak, 1997; Bird et al., 2000; Jensen, 2000; Lu, Crosson, Nadeau, Heilman, Gonzalez-Rothi, Raymer et al., 2002
Reading nouns and/or verbs	Berndt, Mitchum, Haendiges, & Sandson, 1997; Hillis & Caramazza, 1991; Manning & Warrington, 1996; Marshall et al., 1998; Miozzo, Soardi & Cappa, 1994; Pashek, 1998; Renzi & Pellegrino, 1995; Tsapkini, Jarema & Kehayia, 2002
Writing nouns and/or verbs	Daniele, Giustolisi, Silveri, Colosimo & Gainotti, 1994; Hillis & Caramazza, 1991; Hillis, Tuffiash, & Wityk, & Barker, 2002; Jensen, 2000; Miozzo et al., 1994; Rapp & Caramazza, 1998, 2002; Renzi & Pellegrino, 1995
Gesture	Druks & Shallice, 2000; Jensen 2000; McCarthy & Warrington, 1985
Repeating nouns/verbs	Miozzo et al., 1994; Renzi & Pellegrino, 1995; Tsapkini et al., 2002
Retrieving synonyms of verbs	Breedin et al., 1998; Glosser & Donofrio, 2001; Kohn, Lorch & Pearson, 1989; Kremin, 1994; Kohn, Lorch & Pearson, 1989; Laine, Kujala, Niemi & Uusipaikka, 1992
Retrieving antonyms of verbs	Kremin, 1994;
In connected speech/picture description/story completion	Basso, Razzano, Faglioni, Zanobio, 1990; Bastiaanse & Jonkers, 1998; Jonkers & Bastiaanse, 1998; Berndt et al., 1997; Breedin et al., 1998; Kehayia & Jarema, 1991; Kim & Thompson, 2000; Kremin, 1994; Marshall, Chiat, Robson & Pring, 1995/6; Marshall, Pring, Chiat & Robson, 1995/6; Marshall et al., 1998; Pashek, 1998; Thompson et al., 1997; Williams & Canter, 1987; Zingeser & Berndt, 1990
Picture naming Verbs/Nouns/Both	Ardila & Rosselli, 1994; Basso et al., 1990; Bastiaanse, 1991; Bastiaanse & Jonkers, 1998; Bates, Chen, Tzeng, Li & Opie, 1991; Berndt & Haendiges, 2000; Berndt, Mitchum, Haendiges, & Sandson, 1997; Berndt, Haendiges, & Wozniak, 1997; Bird, Howard & Franklin, 2000; Breedin & Martin, 1996; Breedin et al., 1998; Breen & Warrington, 1994; Chen & Bates, 1998; Daniele et al., 1994; Druks & Shallice, 2000; Glosser & Donofrio, 2001; Hillis et al., 2002; Jensen 2000; Jonkers & Bastiaanse, 1996, 1997, 1998; Kambanaros, 2008; Kemmerer & Tranel, 2000; Kim & Thompson, 2000; Kremin, 1986, 1994; Manning & Warrington, 1996; Marshall et al., 1998; Marshall, Chiat, Robson & Pring, 1995/6; Marshall, Pring, Chiat & Robson, 1995/6; McCall, Cox, Shelton, Weinrich, 1997; McCarthy & Warrington, 1985; Miceli, Silveri, Villa, & Caramazza, 1984; Miozzo et al., 1994; Osman-Sagi, 1987; Pashek, 1998; Renzi & Pellegrino, 1995; Thompson et al., 1997; Tsapkini et al., 2002; Williams & Canter, 1987; Zingeser & Berndt, 1990.

Psycholinguistic variables

Moreover, aphasic subjects' error patterns reveal that other variables influence naming accuracy for verbs and nouns regardless of level of breakdown during picture-naming tasks (Caramazza, 1997). Many studies (see Appendix) have demonstrated that visual (picture complexity), semantic (familiarity, operativity) and lexical (age of acquisition [AoA], word frequency, word length) factors also affect the processing of verbs and nouns.

However, each grammatical word class may be influenced by different variables at different stages of the naming process (Colombo & Burani, 2002). In addition, the effect of the different variables can often be linked to the type of errors aphasic patients make when attempting to name a picture. For example, visual complexity and object (or action) familiarity may affect the ease of recognition i.e. influence naming at the "message/pre-semantic" stage. Higher proportions of semantic and phonological errors to particular object names were associated with low familiarity and low visual complexity (Cuetos et al., 2002) while others report that length effects influence naming at the phonological stage but not at the level of semantics (Nickels, 1995; Nickels & Howard, 1995). Similarly, word frequency is postulated to be operative at the phonological output level and generally has no influence in the production of semantic errors (Berndt et al., 1997). In contrast, more recent work has shown word frequency to be important for multiple stages of lexical access (Kittredge, Dell, Verkuilen & Schwartz, 2007) and not only restricted to affecting phonological word processing. Furthermore, the same type of error can occur from damage to different components of the naming process. For example, semantic errors can be a result of breakdown anywhere between lexical-semantic and phonological levels (Hillis & Caramazza, 1995).

Studies have also revealed specific variables that exclusively influence the accurate retrieval of nouns or verbs. For example, instrumentality, name relation and transitivity have been found to influence verb retrieval. It is clear then, that a variety of factors influence naming accuracy in aphasia (Deloche, Hannequin, Dordain, Perrier, Pichard, Quint et al., 1996). Since many of these factors are strongly intercorrelated it is difficult to disentangle their independent effects during naming. For example, both word length and word frequency correlate significantly with age of acquisition revealing that the first words one learns are short and very common, and more resistant to brain injury (see Appendix). Moreover, these findings suggest that no single variable can account for differential subject performance for retrieving verbs and nouns.

Differential Linguistic Properties of Languages

Grammatical word class differences have been investigated in several languages with different underlying forms. Even in the case of languages that are grouped under the same language family such as Indo-European, there are still striking differences between the languages. For example, English and Greek are both Indo-European languages but the latter is highly inflected whereas English is not. However this growing literature on verb-noun breakdown in diverse languages, each with its own language-specific features, has lead to the suggestion that some of the "classical" views reported in English are in need of revision (Roberts, 2001).

Moreover, the largest body of research has been conducted in one language - English. This has fostered premature conclusions in regards to relations between cortical structures and grammar in particular (Slobin, 1991). It has also raised serious questions about generalizing these findings to other languages. For example, grammar, has been shown to break down differently according to the degree of inflection in a language (Bates et al., 1987; Kehayia, Jarema, & Kadzielawa, 1990; Slobin, 1991).

Of interest are the different patterns of impairment in relation to verb/noun retrieval in different languages for both word classes (Bates et al., 1991; Miceli et al., 1988) or within a single grammatical category (Jonkers, 1998; Shapiro et al., 2002; Tsapkini et al., 2002). Findings from these studies highlight two issues. First, that aphasic symptoms in each language can fall into the more generally claimed trends reported in the aphasiology literature. Second, that the findings (of different languages) may reveal strictly language-specific patterns.

Nevertheless, the evidence in the aphasiology literature confirms that verbs and nouns are processed in different ways. Therefore, the dissociation between verbs and nouns remains a consistent finding across languages. This is certainly the case for monolingual aphasic speakers but not much is known about verb-noun dissociations in speakers of two or more languages with aphasia. This issue is explored in detail in the next section.

Bilingual Aphasia

The issue of differential performance on language tasks because of aphasia in bilingual subjects has generated much research. The major thrust of the early clinical literature was to determine which language recovered first and why. The recovery patterns of all published clinical cases of bilingual aphasia have revealed inconclusive findings and according to Green (2005) the incidence of these various recovery patterns is still unknown. Both Fabbro (1999) and Paradis (2001) report that parallel recovery of both languages is the most common phenomenon after a stroke. In parallel recovery both languages are recovered concurrently and to the same degree. This was reported in 40% of all patients studied by Fabbro (1990) and for 61% of patients by Paradis (2001). Better recovery of the native language followed, as reported in 32% of all patients studied. Finally, 28% of patients showed a better recovery of their second language (Fabbro, 1999).

Several factors were considered to affect the recovery process. For example, it was suggested that the native or the last language used prior to the stroke would be the first to recover (Paradis, 1983). This has yet to be proven correct. Nor does it seem that recovery reflected how languages were used or learnt. There are examples of subjects who recovered both languages in a parallel fashion despite learning them in different environments (Sasanuma & Park, 1995). In contrast, others who had acquired both languages in the same environment and were using them daily exhibited a differential recovery (Junque, Vendrell & Vendrell 1995). Moreover, two languages that are structurally similar e.g. Catalan/Spanish and Japanese/Korean have been shown to recover differentially (Junque, Vendrell & Vendrell

1995) while structurally dissimilar languages (Azari/Farsi, English/Farsi) can be recovered in parallel fashion (Nilipour, 1988). It has been argued that recovery pattern types are not related to a preferred language but are linked instead to a control mechanism in the brain. This hypothetical mechanism distributes resources among the various languages spoken (Abutalebi & Green, 2007; Green, 1986). In the case of parallel recovery the control system distributes resources equally to the two languages. In contrast, in the case of differential recovery one language receives more resources than the other and thus recovers sooner.

In addition, other clinical studies of bilingual aphasia have revealed that a bilingual speaker may selectively lose one of his/her languages while the other is spared. Researchers have used this as evidence to suggest that the neural representation of the two languages was differentially organized (Albert & Obler, 1978; Kehayia et al., 1996; Paradis, 1983).

It was hypothesized that the cortical representation of a second language in normal bilingual speakers may differ according to the age it was acquired. In a fMRI study of bilinguals, Kim, Relkin, Lee and Hirsh (1997) reported distinct foci of activation in Broca's area but not Wernicke's for late second language learners. Yet, for early learners both languages resulted in activation in overlapping areas of the brain. In addition, over the past few years a number of neurophysiological and neuroimaging studies have revealed similar cerebral representations of first and second languages both in early and late bilinguals (Chee, Tan, & Thiel, 1999; Hernandez, Martinez & Kohnert, 2000; Illes, Francis, Desmond, Gabrieli, Glover et al, 1999; Klein, Milner, Zatorre, Meyers & Evans, 1995; Klein, Zattore, Milner Meyer & Evans, 1994). However, this view is not shared by all researchers (Kim, Relkin, Lee, Hirsch, 1997; Neville, Mills, & Lawson, 1992; Neville, Coffey, Lawson, Fischer, Emmorey, Bellugi, 1997; Pouratian, Bookheimer, O,Farrell, Sicotte & Cannestra et al., 2000; Weber-Fox & Neville, 1996).

Bilingual Models of Language Processing

One of the most influential models of bilingual lexical processing is the *Revised Hierarchical Model* (Kroll & Stewart 1994) based on findings regarding translation and between-language priming. According to this model, when one learns a second language after childhood, the link between conceptual memory and the native language lexicon is very strong. Thus, the assumption is that both lexical and conceptual connections are active during bilingual word processing, but that the strength of the connections or associations differs according to the relative dominance of L1 over L2 (or vice versa), as well as the language proficiency in L2. As L1 words are strongly linked to conceptual information, translation from L1 to L2 is more likely to trigger conceptual processes, leading to slower processing. Consequently, the model presumes that only L1 processing is conceptually mediated and not L2, especially in late bilinguals.

In contrast, the ability of bilingual speakers to name pictures only in the one (selected) language is interpreted in terms of a language-specific selection account that claims speakers access lexical forms from a language specific subset that can be activated or deactivated in its entirety (De Bot & Schreuder, 1993; Green, 1986, 1993; 1998; Paradis, 1989). It is assumed that a bilingual individual can produce words only in the language in which he or she intends to speak because the activation level of lexical representations in that language is higher than the activation level of language(s) not chosen for production

Grosjean (1985, 1997) describes this activating/deactivating process of the two languages during speech as allowing the bilingual speaker to perform in different language modes: the monolingual mode where one language is exclusively spoken as the other is partially deactivated and the bilingual mode where one language is adopted as the base language and the second language serves as the "guest" language and is used when code-switching or language mixing. Thus, both languages are active but the base one is more strongly activated.

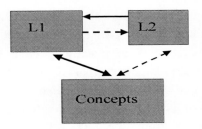

Revised Hierarchical Model

Figure 2. The Revised Hierarchical Model of bilingual lexical-semantic representation.

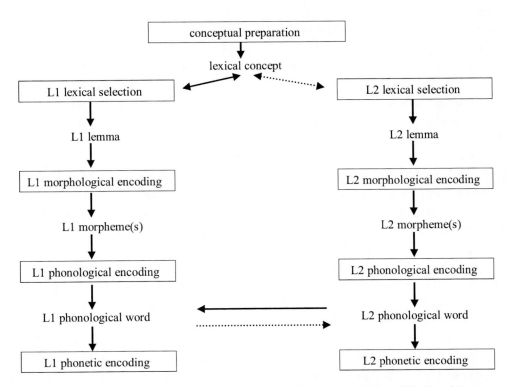

Figure 3. A bilingual model of word production based on Levelt et al., 1999 and Kroll and Stewart, 1994. Important elements are: L1 is more conceptually mediated than L2, the asymmetry of L1-L2 and L2-L1 translation and priming effects, and the language-specific nature of lexical selection, and morphological -, phonological -, and phonetic encoding.

Figure 3 as proposed by Kambanaros and van Steenbrugge (2006) represents a combination of Levelt's serial model for word processing (Levelt, 1989; Levelt, Roelofs & Meyer, 1999) and the RHM (Kroll & Stewart, 1994) in which lexical processing is organised in three relatively distinct levels: conceptual, syntactic and morpho-phonological level (see Levelt et al., 1999 for a detailed description). The bilingual model for word retrieval and production is based on a number of assumptions: (1) the first stages of the model, conceptual preparation and accessing the lexical concept are non-language specific; whereas (2) the other stages, lexical selection or lemma activation, morphological -, phonological – and phonetic encoding are language specific; (3) L1 is more conceptually mediated than L2 represented by the stronger link between lexical concept and L1 lexical selection; and (4) asymmetric translation effects with faster L2-L1 translation represented by the stronger link from L2 to L1 than to L1 to L2 [N.B. asymmetric priming effects have been found in opposite direction, with a larger priming effect from L1 to L2 than from L2 to L1, leading to the assumptions that L1 is more conceptually mediated than L2 (Keatley, Spinks & de Gelder, 1994). Articulation is not included in the model because of the variable speech output in bilingual individuals ranging from speaking with a heavy accent to native-like pronunciation of their two languages.

A prominent feature of the model is that only words of the target language are in competition and retrieved during lexical selection (Costa, Miozzo & Caramazza, 1999). This is congruent with Levelt et al.'s assumption that lexical selection and lemma activation must be language specific because of the language-specific nature of the grammatical information contained in lemmas (Levelt et al., 1999). Language specificity must also be preserved further down in the model because of language-specific morphological, phonological and rule systems of different languages.

Lexical selection or lemma activation is an essential element of the model. An activated concept spreads some of its activation to the corresponding lemma and is selected when its activation level equals or exceeds the ratio of its activation to the sum activation of all (competing) lemmas. The syntactic or grammatical information of the lemma becomes available upon its selection and activation. Noun lemmas contain information about grammatical properties like their syntactic category (e.g., + noun), gender and number, whereas verb lemmas contain information about syntactic category (e.g., + verb), person, tense and mood. Syntactic category (noun, verb, adjective, etc.) is a property at lemma level according to Levelt et al., (1999).

Lemma retrieval is always part of word production, independent of the syntactic context or the task. Only selected lemmas will become activated during morpho-phonological encoding. Semantic substitutions are considered to result from spreading activation within the conceptual network that in turn leads to a failure in lemma selection or the activation of two lemmas at the same time which may explain the syntactic constraint of substitution errors in normal speakers, that is, substitution errors within the same syntactic category (Levelt et al., 1999). Overall, word processing can be affected at three relatively distinct stages: during lexical selection, during lemma activation or when activating the (morpho-) phonological word forms, but the level of breakdown is not always immediately apparent.

The above findings are linked to the key issue in bilingual word processing, namely whether word forms of each language are represented in one common lexicon and semantic memory system or in two separate lexicons or semantic memory systems (Altenberg & Cairns, 1983). This issue has been the subject of much research and debate. Currently, two predominant but conflicting theories exist.

The first theory is that concepts are stored in a common, non-language-specific semantic system but words within the lexicon form two subsets (de Bot, 1992; Paradis, 1989, 2000) each containing language-specific syntactic, morphological and phonological information. Additional evidence to support the hypothesis that the two languages of a bilingual access a common semantic system comes from neuroimaging studies (Illes, Francis, Desmond, Gabrieli, Glover et al, 1999). The second theory draws on the similarities between bilinguals and monolinguals by proposing a single lexical system for bilinguals and monolinguals particularly in the domain of morphology (Kirsner, Lalor & Hird, 1993; Lalor & Kirsner, 2001). Lalor and Kirsner recently claimed the following:

> …"boundaries in the bilingual system are not governed by language but by morphology, that is by similarity in form and meaning"(p.1048)

The above differences in the age and manner of learning and using language by bilingual speakers have been linked to two distinct kinds of memory systems, each with a specific language capacity, that are neurofunctionally and anatomically different and that can be differentially affected by brain injury (Paradis, 1995; Ullman, 2001). More specifically, it is hypothesized that a second language when learned formally or consciously in an educational setting is subserved primarily by declarative memory (Fabbro, 2001, Paradis, 1995, 2000 Ullman, 2001). The declarative memory system, also known as explicit memory, encompasses the semantic (knowledge about facts) and episodic (knowledge of events) memory systems and is represented in medial temporal and parietal neocortical regions including the hippocampus and related structures. Ullman (2001) defines the declarative memory system as "an associative memory that underlies stored knowledge about words including their sounds, their meanings, and other memorized information" (p.106). Alternatively, this is described as explicit metalinguistic knowledge (Paradis, 2000).

On the other hand, if the second language is acquired informally, that is incidentally, as is the case with the native language, it is sustained essentially by procedural memory and is used automatically. This memory system is synonymous with implicit memory and has been implicated in the learning of novel motor and cognitive skills. It appears to be controlled by frontal/basal ganglia structures. Ullman (2001) states that the "learning and use of aspects of a symbol manipulating grammar, across grammatical subdomains, including syntax, non-lexical semantics, morphology and phonology " (p.107) is posited by procedural memory. Alternatively this is described as implicit linguistic competence (Paradis 2000).

In brief, the declarative/procedural model hypothesizes that the declarative memory system underlies the learning, representation, and use of aspects of lexical knowledge while the procedural memory system underlies the learning, representation, and use of aspects of grammatical knowledge. Moreover, this hypothesis was also applied to the area of late second language acquisition that is when L2 is acquired after late childhood or puberty with the presupposition that the two memory systems (i.e. declarative/procedural) tend to play a somewhat different role in later-acquired second (and subsequent) languages. Later exposure to language may impair the ability of the procedural memory system to learn or compute aspects of grammar so that grammatical computational rules in the second language are more dependent upon declarative or lexical memory than on the procedural memory system (Ullman, 2001).

In addition, it is claimed that the amount of practice or degree of L2 use also affects both grammatical proficiency and the degree of dependence on procedural memory for grammatical computations, mainly that the less a bilingual speaker uses his/her L2 the larger the degree of dependence on declarative memory for grammatical computations (Paradis, 1995; Ullman, 2001). This prediction with respect to L1 and L2 grammatical language processing is supported by functional imaging studies (Dehaene, Dupoux, Mehler, Cohen, Paulesu et al., 1997; Perani, Paulesu, Galles, Dupoux, Dehaene et al., 1998) and lesion studies (Fabbro, 1999). In sum, a more recent neurolinguistic theory as proposed by Paradis (2004) and the account of L2 representation as proposed by Ullman, (2005) rely on the notion of two distinct memory systems. Both proposals agree that words are represented in one system and implicit grammatical competence in another and there are differences in the the the representation of syntax in L2 compared to L1.

Finally, research in the area of bilingualism has increased over the last decade primarily in the area of psycholinguistics. This research, including research in bilingual aphasia, has led to contradictory findings, much like the outcomes observed in monolingual aphasia. It has been suggested that many of the conflicting outcomes could have been avoided if researchers had taken into account differences between monolinguals and bilinguals by becoming more aware of how bilingual subjects function in varying linguistic environments. Furthermore, information regarding when the languages were acquired, how they were learned, what language skills were acquired (listening, speaking, reading, writing) and how the languages were used on a daily basis affects the state of bilingualism in any individual (Grosjean, 1997, 1998). Specifically, in subjects with bilingual aphasia this information is of paramount importance when testing language abilities and interpreting the findings (Ullman, 1999; 2001).

Verb and Noun Processing in Bilingual Aphasia

Research to date on verb and noun processing in bilingual aphasia is sparse. This area should not be considered a separate field of inquiry from its monolingual counterpart but a part of research that seeks to understand language per se (De Bot, 1992). [4]

An interesting aspect of studying bilingual aphasia is investigating whether linguistic and grammatical distinctions such as the grammatical distinction between nouns and verbs, are language specific or not. If not, that is, if similar processing differences are observed during noun and verb processing in either language, one could conclude that nouns and verbs of

---

[4] In this review of the literature only a few studies were found using picture naming as the method to assess naming performance in bilingual aphasia. These studies focused on concrete noun retrieval with one aim: to demonstrate differential naming performance in the two languages spoken by the aphasic individual(s) (Kremin & De Agostini, 1995; Junque, Vendrell, Vendrell, 1989, 1995; Stadie, Springer, de Bleser & Burk, 1995).

both languages are processed in a similar manner by the same cortical and subcortical areas in the brain. In other words, neurophysiological processes involved in word processing must be primarily affected by the grammatical category of the word rather than the language in which the word is presented.

Six studies have been found in the literature investigating verb and noun differences in bilingual patients; three studies involve patients with a fluent and/or anomic aphasia resulting from a left hemisphere lesion, one study reports noun-verb dissociations in an individual with Alzheimers Disease and the other following onset of Primary Progressive Aphasia. A summary of the studies describing grammatical word class effects in language-impaired bilingual adults is presented in Table 2.

In the first study, a single case of a trilingual aphasic subject with word-finding difficulties in all three languages was reported. However, verb and noun retrieval were probed using picture naming only in the subject's second language, Italian. Both action and object words were retrieved equally well (97% and 93% respectively).

In the second study, Sasanuma and Park (1995) also assessed naming in a fluent aphasic male in two languages, Korean (L1) and Japanese (L2), using an aphasia test in each language across the four modalities (auditory, reading, oral production and writing). They described greater word retrieval difficulties in L2 compared to L1 for both verbs and nouns in picture naming and conversation.

In the study by Hernandez et al., (2006) a grammatical class dissociation was reported in a patient with Alzheimer's disease (AD) who presented with a significantly worse performance in retrieving nouns compared to verbs on naming tasks in both Catalan (L1) and Spanish (L2) despite good comprehension for both word classes across languages.

Similarly, in the study by Hernandez et al., (2008) a grammatical class deficit was reported in a bilingual Spanish (L1) and Catalan (L2) patient with Primary Progressive Aphasia (PPA) who presented with more difficulties in naming verbs compared to nouns on both spoken and written naming tasks in both languages. The patient's naming performances and error types for verbs were similar across both languages but with a worse performance in L2.

In the above two studies, grammatical class deficits are reported in two patients with different underlying brain pathology that excludes stroke or a focal lesion. Both AD and PPA are progressive and degenerative diseases, the latter of unknown etiology, that involve more extensive cerebral damage. In this case, it could prove difficult to tease out deficits to different types of semantic information (e.g. action and object names) and impairments to lexical networks in the brain. Furthermore, grammatical class effects are reported in two languages (Spanish and Catalan) of similar morphosyntactic complexity and overlapping phonological properties. This raises two questions namely a) how grammatical word class properties are stored and retrieved in typologically similar languages and b) the relationship between lexical and syntactic deficits in typologically similar languages.

Poncelet et al., (2007) asked bilingual aphasic participants to name pictures of actions and objects (from the Action and Object naming battery: Druks & Masterson, 2000) both in L1 and L2 (at least one week apart). All three patients retrieved object names significantly better than action names in both their languages with a better performance in their L1. Also, one subject (PJ) had memory and attention deficits because of cerebral anoxia thus making it difficult to decifer the (detrimental) role of executive functions (memory, attention) on picture naming for grammatical word classes.

In the study by Kambanaros and van Steenbrugge (2006), potential selective noun and/or verb processing deficits were investigated in bilingual individuals with anomic aphasia, to determine whether or not any specific noun or verb impairments were confined to their first language (Greek) or could also be found in their second language (English). The findings revealed that verbs were significantly more difficult to retrieve than nouns when naming pictures of actions and objects, irrespective of what language was used by the bilingual aphasic speakers. The findings were not affected by overall (residual) language proficiency in the two languages, nor by well known factors, such as word frequency and imageability.

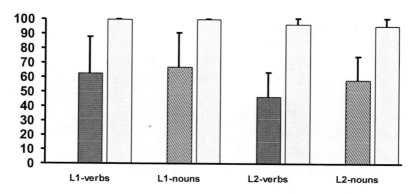

Figure 4. Mean percentages and Standard Deviations for object/noun naming and action/verb naming in L1 and L2 in the aphasic (patterned bars) and non-brain injured individuals.

Interestingly, there was little individual variation across the bilingual participants with anomic aphasia. Luzzatti et al., (2002) showed a significant degree of individual variability across the individuals with anomic aphasia in their study. This variability of performance and underlying deficit was echoed by Shapiro and Caramazza (2001) who stressed that there might be no single deficit underlying the disorder. The individual variability was relatively small in the current study. All twelve aphasic subjects showed better noun than verb retrieval in Greek, whereas nine subjects also showed better noun than verb production in English. Of the remaining three anomic individuals, one showed the reverse pattern, whereas the other two showed an equal ability in noun and verb production in English.

Moreover, instrumentality and name-relation individually influenced verb processing in the group under investigation by Kambanaros and van Steenbrugge (2006) similarly in L1 and L2, and therefore no language-specific effects were demonstrated. Bilingual aphasic subjects found instrumental verbs significantly easier to retrieve than non-instrumental verbs during naming in their native (Greek) and second language (English), demonstrating a cross-linguistic effect of instrumentality on verb retrieval.

Grammatical Word Class Breakdown in Bilingual Aphasia

Only six studies (see Table 2) were found that examine evidence for the representation and processing of verbs and nouns in the two languages of bilingual aphasic individuals with anomia i.e. word finding difficulties. Four studies involved the description of single cases (Kremin & De Agostini, 1995; Sasanuma & Park, 1995; Hernandez, et al., 2006; Hernandez, et al., 2008) while the remaining two studies involved small groups of three (Poncelet, et al., 2007) and twelve bilingual patients (Kambanaros & van Steenbrugge, 2006). Across all studies, 19 bilingual aphasic individuals took part, 13 males and 6 females, and all were assessed using picture naming tasks involving action and object names in a total of 11 different languages (Bergasmac, Catalan, English, French, German, Greek, Italian, Japanese, Korean, Spanish, Turkish). However, only in three studies are patients typically anomic aphasic as a result of a cerebrovascular accident (CVA) in the left hemisphere (Kambanaros & van Steenbrugge, 2006; Poncelet et al., 2007; Sasanuma & Park, 1995). Furthermore, patterns of second language acquisition in the bilingual aphasic patients in the above-mentioned studies differed with some individuals acquiring L2 in early adulthood upon migration to the L2 country (Kambanaros & van Steenbrugge, 2006) while others were early bilinguals (Hernandez et al., 2007; 2008; Kremin & De Agostini, 1995; Sasanuma & Park, 1995). However all bilingual aphasic patients were reported to be proficient users of their L2 prior to the onset of aphasia. In addition, the recovery patterns following brain injury revealed a differential recovery of the two languages with a better preserved L1 in most cases (Hernandez et al., 2006; Kambanaros & van Steenbrugge, 2006; Kremin & De Agostini, 1995; Sasanuma & Park, 1995).

The results from the studies (see Table 2) in relation to verb-noun breakdown and patterns of performance in bilingual aphasic speakers reveal four distinct findings:

1. No differences in retrieving the names of objects or actions in L1 and L2 (Kremin & De Agostini, 1995; Sasanuma & Park, 1995);
2. A significant dissociation between verbs and nouns with object names more difficult to retrieve than action names in L1 and L2 in anomic aphasia (Hernandez et al., 2006);
3. A significant dissociation between verbs and nouns with action names more difficult to retrieve than object names in L1 and L2 in agrammatism (Hernandez et al., 2008)
4. A significant dissociation between verbs and nouns with action names more difficult to retrieve than object names in L1 and L2 in anomic aphasia (Kambanaros & van Steenbrugge, 2006; Poncelet et al., 2007).

The first finding based on the results from the earlier studies investigating verb-noun production in bilingual aphasia do not reveal a grammatical class effect as observed with many other monolingual (anomic) patients (e.g., Basso et al., 1990; Luzzatti et al., 2002). Kremin and De Agostini claimed that their finding substantiated two earlier assumptions from the monolingual literature: that action naming is not necessarily significantly preserved in anomia (Basso et al., 1990) and that there is no direct relationship between selective verb-noun impairments and aphasia type (Kremin & Basso, 1993). However, this study is somewhat flawed.

Table 2. A summary of the studies describing grammatical word class effects in language-impaired bilingual adults.

Study	Participants	Gender	Diagnosis	Languages	Grammatical word class differences	Methodology
1.Kremin & De Agostini (1995)	1	female	lesion in the left hemisphere of unknown etiology	Bergamac (L1) Italian (L2) German (L3)	Nouns = Verbs *Grammatical class differences tested in L2 only.	picture naming
2. Sasanuma & Park (1995)	1	male	Left CVA (MCA)	Korean (L1) Japanese (L2)	?Nouns = Verbs	picture naming & spontaneous speech
3. Kambanaros & van Steenbrugge (2006)	12	8 males 4 females	anomic aphasia (Left CVAs)	Greek (L1) English (L2)	Nouns > Verbs	picture naming
4. Hernandez, Costa, Sebastian-Galles, Juncadella, & Rene (2006)	1	female	anomic (BDAE-Cookie theft picture) Alzheimer's disease	Catalan (L1) Spanish (L2)	Nouns < Verbs	picture naming
5. Poncelet, Majerus, Raman, Warinbaire & Weekes (2007)	3	males	Anomic aphasia (Left CVAs) for 2 patients Cerebral anoxia for 1 patient	Turkish (L1)-English (L2) (for one patient) German (L1)-French (L2) (for two patients)	Nouns > Verbs	picture naming
6. Hernandez, Cano, Costa, Sebastian-Galles, Juncadella & Gascon-Bayarri, (2008)	1	male	non-fluent agrammatic (BDAE-Cookie theft picture) Primary Progressive Aphasia	Spanish (L1) Catalan (L2)	Nouns > Verbs	picture naming: verbal and written

Key: CVA= Cerebrovascular accident, MCA=Middle Cerebral Artery, BDAE=Boston Diagnostic Aphasia Examination

First, the conclusions are based on the results of one subject who was assessed in only one of her three languages, Italian. The subject lived in Italy yet used all three languages prior to her illness for different purposes (employment, with family etc) on a daily basis. Therefore, results from one language only are not representative of the subjects' verb-noun processing abilities in the other two languages, especially in this case where the subjects' linguistic abilities differed across her three languages after her illness. Her first language, Bergamasc, was better preserved than Italian and her third language, German, was the most impaired.

Second, the subject was not a "typical" aphasic individual since her lesion in the left hemisphere was of unknown etiology and not related to stroke or neurological impairment. She presented with anomia after many years of epilepsy followed by removal of a tumour from the right temporal lobe. Third, the assessment materials were based on action and object pictures originally constructed in French, a language with a different deep structure to Italian. Finally, the researchers controlled only for frequency (high frequency) of the test items. It is possible then that the subject's high action and object naming scores were the result of a frequency effect (i.e. words of high frequency are easier to retrieve).

In the second study supporting pattern one, Sasanuma and Park (1995) failed to describe the test items or the results in each grammatical category (verbs/nouns) for either language. Therefore, their results are more in tune with findings from language recovery studies (i.e. which language recovers better and why) rather than grammatical word class processing.

Consequently, the above findings provide little useful information in relation to verb-noun dissociations in bilingual aphasia. This is because in the latter study grammatical word class processing was not of specific interest and in the first study, key methodological and conceptual issues related to bilingualism were not taken into consideration. For example, Kremin and De Agostini, (1995) reported verb-noun performance in one language and ignored the other(s) and in by doing so adopted the fractionalized view of bilingualism[5] (Grosjean, 1985; 1989).

A number of studies have revealed selective noun impairments in monolingual aphasic subjects with anomia in different languages (Berndt et al., 1997; Breen & Warrington, 1994; Damasio & Tranel, 1993; Daniele et al., 1994; De Renzi & Di Pellegrino, 1995; Miozzo, Soardi & Cappa, 1994; Silveri & Di Betta, 1997; Zingeser & Berndt, 1988, 1990). Patients with anomia are considered to have deficits in accessing the phonological information/representation of a target word (Kay & Ellis, 1987). In this case, noun retrieval breakdown is assumed at the level of the word form. Further additional evidence of noun-verb dissociations has come from studies involving individuals with semantic dementia (Bird, Lambon Ralph, Patterson & Hodges, 2000; Breedin, Saffran & Coslett, 1994; Schwartz, Marin & Saffran 1979). In the bilingual context, Hernandez et al., (2006) attribute the significant difficulty their bilingual anomic patient with Alzheimers Disease has in retrieving object names compared to action names to an impairment at the lexeme level for nouns (see lexical account).

In addition Hernandez et al., (2008) argue that the verb retrieval deficit in their bilingual patient with agrammatic aphasia (PPA) is due to damage at the level of the lexicon.

---

[5] A bilingual functions as two (or more) separate monolinguals, with no influence of one language on another.

Specifically, an overall reduced ability to access verbs but preserved ability to name nouns is associated with agrammatism, often found in Broca's or non-fluent aphasia, as a result of lesions in the frontal areas of the left cerebral hemisphere. The difficulties agrammatic subjects encounter accessing verbs is often attributed to a breakdown at the level of the lemma. It is assumed that subjects with agrammatism may have grammatical difficulties because of an impaired grammatical encoder (Bastiaanse, 1991) or a syntactic deficit (Zingeser & Berndt, 1990) related to their difficulties in producing grammatically correct sentences (Saffran, Schwartz & Marin, 1980; Saffran, 1982), and/or problems at the morphological level (Caramazza & Berndt, 1985). However, verb deficits can arise at the level of the phonological word form if one assumes that verbs and nouns are stored in independent subsystems, possibly with distinct neural substrates and pathways for retrieving the phonological form. This conclusion is often obtained in the absence of major syntactic and semantic deficits (see lexical account).

The last finding of a better noun than verb retrieval (Kambanaros & van Steenbrugge, 2006; Poncelet et al., 2007) is at odds with previous findings of (i)specific noun retrieval problems in anomic patients who speak one language (eg., Miceli et al., 1984; Zingeser & Berndt, 1990; Laiacona & Caramazza, 2004; Shapiro et al., 2000), or two (Hernandez et al., 2006) and (ii) studies in which no verb-noun dissociation was found in monolingual and bilingual anomic patients (see above). The finding provides further evidence that a difficulty retrieving verbs is not necessarily restricted to agrammatism (Berndt et al., 1997; Caramazza & Hillis, 1991). The strong advantage for noun production in bilingual aphasic subjects with anomia is more in line with a processing account of the noun-verb dichotomy, namely that verbs are overall more difficult to retrieve than nouns. This finding is congruent with earlier studies in which verbs were also found to be more difficult to retrieve than nouns in monolingual anomic speakers of different languages (Bastiaanse & Jonkers, 1998; Berndt & Haendiges, 2000; Berndt et al, 1997; Jonkers, 1998; Jonkers & Bastiaanse, 1996, 1998; Kohn et al., 1989; Luzzatti et al., 2002; McCann & Edwards, 2002; Williams & Canter, 1987). The fact that the verb-noun dissociation was observed in both the languages spoken by the bilingual subjects suggests that this dissociation is not specific to a particular language, but is likely to arise from more universal conceptual and/or linguistic characteristics that differentiate words belonging to the two grammatical categories.

Level of Verb-noun Breakdown in Bilingual Anomic Aphasia

Psycholinguistic explanation

Following on from the model presented in Figure 3, the verb-retrieval impairment may be due to a breakdown at any of the four relatively discrete word processing levels: (1) the activation of the conceptual-semantic representation for the action, i.e., the lexical-semantic account; (2) the activation and selection of the specific verb lemma, i.e., the lexical-grammatical account; (3) the activation of the morphological representation; or (4) the activation of the phonological representation. The first two accounts are based on greater complexity in the underlying representations of verbs compared to those of nouns, in terms of their conceptual-semantic or syntactic representation respectively. The last two explanations are based on the assumption of a selective deficit in components of a lexicon subdivided according to grammatical distinctions between the classes of words.

The finding of a verb-noun dissociation in both languages could be interpreted as supporting the hypothesis that verbs are more conceptually complex than nouns which may be particularly evident during naming (e.g., Bird et al., 2000; Kohn et al., 1989; Williams & Canter, 1987). For instance, most action verbs carry an implicit agent initiating the action. The agent of each verb was explicitly present in the naming task, i.e. present in the photograph displaying the action to be named. In other words, the verb-noun dissociation may result from a deficit at conceptual-semantic level before language-specific lexical retrieval processes are initiated. This has lead to the view that noun/verb effects result from differences within the semantic representations of the two word classes. Under assumptions of spreading activation, it is possible that verbs compared to nouns have a broader set of activated competitors at the level of the lemma.

Poncelet et al., (2007) attributed the verb breakdown in their bilingual anomic patients to the fact that action names may be more vulnerable to brain damage given the greater semantic complexity of verbs compared to nouns. The authors reported that picture imageability had a significant facilitatory effect on naming performances for object names than for action names. It has been claimed (Bird et al., 2000) that verb-noun dissociations result from a selective impairment of perceptual or functional semantic features. However comprehension of action and object names was not reported making it difficult to determine if patients had similar difficulties or pattern of performance in comprehension.

In the study by Kambanaros & van Steenbrugge (2006), where comprehension performances are reported, the bilingual anomic individuals did not show a similar dissociation in their comprehension of the same target nouns and verbs, In fact, they showed little difficulty comprehending the content words of either language. The specific verb impairment is, therefore, unlikely to result from a central deficit at this early stage of word retrieval, especially since the same target nouns and verbs were used in both languages. This argument is further strengthened by the finding that the verb-noun dissociation was unaffected by the difference in overall L1 and L2 proficiency in the anomic individuals (and in the non-brain injured control group) (cf Kambanaros & van Steenbrugge, 2006).

The specific verb impairment in the above-mentioned study may also have resulted from an underlying deficit at lemma level, during the activation of the verb (and noun) lemma given that verb lemmas convey greater grammatical complexity than noun lemmas. This conclusion is somewhat supported by the high number of semantic substitutions in the naming errors, possibly due to the simultaneous activation of more than one lemma for the target verb and/or noun (cf Kambanaros & van Steenbrugge, 2006). The impairment at the level of the lemma may make it more difficult for the aphasic individual to select the single, correct target verb. Semantic substitutions are considered to result from spreading activation within the conceptual network that in turn leads to a failure in lemma selection because of either the simultaneous activation of two or more concepts (conceptual intrusion) or the activation of two or more lemmas at the same time (associative intrusion/word associations) which may explain the syntactic constraint of substitution errors, that is substitution errors within the same syntactic category (Levelt, 1989; Levelt et al., 1999). In addition, semantic errors have also been reported as the most prominent error type in other verb retrieval studies involving (monolingual) anomic individuals (Bastiaanse, 1991; Berndt, Burton et al., 2002; Berndt, Mitchum et al., 1997; Jonkers, 1998).

With regards to semantic errors being more prevalent in L2, this may stem from bilingual aphasic individuals' difficulties directly accessing L2 conceptual information. According to the Revised Hierarchical Model RHM (Kroll & Stewart, 1994), there is a stronger connection between concept information and L1 especially in late bilinguals, even when bilingual subjects are proficient in the second language (see Figure 2). This does not necessarily mean that late bilingual individuals do not have immediate access to the meaning of L2 words. It may indicate that they do not have access to additional conceptual information, possibly because of limited or reduced spreading activation through the semantic or conceptual network when processing L2 words.

Since lemmas are supposedly shared in production and comprehension (Levelt et al., 1999), one would expect the bilingual individuals to demonstrate the same pattern in comprehension i.e., more difficulty with verbs compared to nouns in L1 and L2. However, this was not the case in the study by Kambanaros and van Steenbrugge (2006). All bilingual aphasic patients demonstrated relatively intact (but not perfect) comprehension of verb meanings in either language. This finding supports the assumption that comprehension tasks may not be sensitive enough to discover minimal semantic and or lexical/syntactic deficits (Berndt et al., 1997; Gainotti et al., 1995; Sacchett & Humphries, 1992).

On the other hand, there is also a strong argument against the assumption of a specific verb impairment at the level of the lemma. Berndt and colleagues (Berndt et al., 1997; Berndt et al., 2002; Berndt & Haendiges, 2000) pointed out that any specific verb lemma deficit should also lead to verb retrieval problems during sentence construction and in spontaneous speech. Such verb retrieval problems were not evident in this group of bilingual anomic individuals as they did not show any substantial verb retrieval impairment in their spontaneous speech, especially not in L1(Greek) (Kambanaros, 2007, in press). The second argument is that few verb-noun or noun-verb substitutions were recorded during naming in both languages, suggesting that lemma information about grammatical word category could be successfully retrieved (cf Kambanaros & van Steenbrugge, 2006).

The effects of instrumentality (a conceptual and lemma feature) and Verb-noun name relation (a phonological feature) on action naming were also investigated in this group of bilingual individuals with anomic aphasia and a non-brain injured, bilingual control group. As expected, there were no significant differences between the aphasic and non-brain injured group in L1 and L2 comprehension of the verbs used in the action naming task, nor did either group show any effect of Instrumentality or Verb-noun relation in L1 and L2 word comprehension.

Instrumentality had a significant, positive effect on action naming in the bilingual individuals with anomic aphasia, in that instrumental verbs were easier to retrieve than non-instrumental verbs in both languages. On the other hand, Verb-noun name relation had a negative effect on verb naming in the same individuals in both languages, but the effect was significant in L2 (English) only. Thus, (English) instrumental verbs with a noun name relation were more difficult to retrieve than the instrumental verbs without a noun name relation. Both aphasic and non-brain injured bilingual individuals showed more difficulty producing verbs in their second language (English) than in their first language (Greek), but naming in the non-brain injured bilingual individuals was not affected by the effects of instrumentality and verb-noun relation who showed ceiling effects on each task (cf Kambanaros & van Steenbrugge, 2006).

The finding of a positive effect of instrumentality is congruent with earlier findings in a number of studies in which monolingual individuals with anomic aphasia were also found to have less difficulty retrieving instrumental than non-instrumental actions (e.g., Breedin et al., 1998, 1999; Jonkers, 1998; Jonkers & Bastiaanse, 1996). Breedin and others (1998, 1999) suggest that verb retrieval can be facilitated by semantic complexity in some individuals with aphasia. Given that instrumental verbs are semantically more complex than non-instrumental verbs, semantic complexity might have facilitated the retrieval of instrumental verbs (Breedin et al., 1998, 1999). In other words, the facilitating effect might be due to the automatic co-activation of the instrumental noun lemma whenever an instrumental verb lemma is activated (Bastiaanse, 1991; Jonkers, 1998). Additional support for the latter comes from a word-priming study in which Ferretti, McRae and Hatherall (2001) found that instrumental verbs presented in isolation primed the related instruments (nouns) in non-brain injured adults. For example, reading the verb 'stirred' activated information about the instrumental noun 'spoon'. In contrast, non-instrumental verb lemmas do not contain semantic/conceptual information about the related noun (e.g., to sleep – bed), and therefore there is no co-activation of the associated noun. Although such co-activation is theoretically possible during lexical selection and lemma activation, it will not directly facilitate verb retrieval because there is no direct, lemma-bound relationship between the conceptual representation of the verb and the noun. The bilingual individuals with anomic aphasia may have found the less complex, non-instrumental verbs more difficult to retrieve, because non-instrumental verbs are semantically under-specified compared to instrumental verbs (Breedin et al., 1996; 1998; 1999). The simultaneous activation of the related lemma of the instrumental noun might also have facilitated retrieval of the word form of the target instrumental verb during a Tip-of-the-Tongue (TOT) state in which the individual is aware of the (temporary) problem of the failure to activate the correct word form. Given that instrumentality is a conceptual feature of the Greek and English language, it is not surprising that the effect of instrumentality was observed in both languages spoken by the bilingual individuals with anomic aphasia. The finding was not confounded by verb-noun name relation as only instrumental verbs without a noun name relation were used in the comparison.

On the other hand, the effect of verb-noun name relation was only confined to L2 (English). Bilingual individuals with anomic aphasia (but not the normal controls) experienced more difficulty retrieving L2 instrumental verbs with a noun name relation than L2 instrumental verbs without a noun name relation. No effect of verb-noun name relation was found in L1 (Greek). There were no significant differences between L1 instrumental verbs with or without a noun name relation. The findings in the native language are contradictory to earlier findings of a positive effect of Verb-noun name relation (Kemmerer & Tranel; 2000; Kremin, 1994), but are congruent with earlier results of no significant differences in monolingual individuals with anomic aphasia (Jonkers, 1998; Jonkers & Bastiaanse, 1996). The negative effect of Verb-noun name relation in L2 (English) was unforeseen as the opposite effect was expected based on earlier findings in English (Breedin et al, 1999; Kemmerer & Tranel, 2000). However, the latter study does not include specific information about aphasia syndrome and a different task (sentence completion) was used in the former study, making a direct comparison between the results of these two studies and the current study virtually impossible. Moreover, a similar finding has been reported previously by Bastiaanse (1991), in that one of the two anomic participants (An.2) also showed better performance for non-name related instrumental verbs.

Returning to the model in Figure 3, the specific verb impairment in the bilingual individuals with anomic aphasia in the Kambanaros & van Steenbrugge study might have arisen at the level of morphological processing, given that a substantial number of the Greek verbs included in the study had a more complex morphological structure [root+affix] and [root + affix + affix] than the Greek nouns [root + affix]. However, the relatively small number of suffixation-errors in Greek and omissions in English only render this unlikely (cf Kambanaros & van Steenbrugge, 2006). The anomic individuals made also very few phonological errors (cf Kambanaros & van Steenbrugge, 2006) which does not seem to support the assumption of a specific phonological processing difficulty. However, it is possible that *access* to the (morpho-) phonological representation of the target words is affected in (bilingual) anomic aphasia, leaving the actual morpho-phonological representations intact (Bastiaanse & Jonkers, 1998; Jonkers, 1998; Tsapkini et al., 2002).

In sum, Kambanaros and van Steenbrugge suggested that the specific verb impairment in both languages was most likely the result of a greater difficulty accessing the (morpho-) phonological representation or lexemes of verbs. The similarity of the verb impairment in the two languages as well as the similarity in the types of naming errors observed suggested the same level of breakdown when producing words in either language (see Kambanaros & van Steenbrugge, 2006). Although the naming deficit was more severe in the second language of the bilingual anomic patients, the findings could not be attributed to their overall lower L2 proficiency. As the verb-noun dissociation was evident in L1 (Greek), and L2 (English) it is clear that this finding is non-language specific and unrelated to differences in the underlying linguistic features of the two languages. Overall, the results suggested a genuine non-language specific difference in accessing/retrieving verbs and nouns during single word and this dissociation was relatively independent of subjects' residual L1 and L2 language proficiency

However, the bilingual aphasic subjects had little difficulty producing verbs in connected speech in either language (Kambanaros, 2007). This finding demonstrated that a verb production difficulty in single word production (particularly action/verb confrontation naming) for bilingual anomic subjects did not co-occur with verb production difficulties in spontaneous speech (Kambanaros, in press). This has also been reported for monolingual anomic/fluent aphasic speakers of English (Bastiaanse et al., 1996; Goodglass, et al., 1993), Dutch (Bastiaanse et al., 1996; Bastiaanse & Jonkers, 1998) and Hungarian (Bastiaanse et al., 1996). However, subjects did produce significantly more verbs in their native language (Greek) and they also produced a significantly smaller variety (diversity) of verbs in their second language (English), revealing access (presumably) to a reduced range of verbs, possibly because of less conceptually mediated word processing in L2. Again, this finding lends support for the RHM (Kroll & Stewart, 1994).

Overall, the main finding that verbs are more difficult to retrieve than nouns in this group of bilingual anomic aphasic speakers of Greek and English seems to lend support to the following three assumptions. First, verb retrieval impairments are not confined to agrammatism and linked to frontal or pre-frontal lesions. Second, verbs are inherently more difficult to produce than nouns because of more abstract differentiations in their underlying semantic/thematic or syntactic structure. Third, the verb deficit follows a breakdown of the verb-retrieval process at the morpho-phonological stage of lexical representation.

The prevailing view of anomic aphasia is that anomic individuals have difficulty retrieving the phonological form (the 'lexeme') of the target word (Goodglass, 1993), i.e., their difficulty arises at the morpho-phonological level. As discussed previously, the syntactic information of the target word is also important during the activation of its morphological representation. Furthermore, Edwards (2002) defined the breakdown in fluent (Wernicke's) aphasia as occurring "in accessing lexical items which in turn arise from either semantically based problems or from problems in phonological representation" (p. 249-250). Bachoud-Lévi and Dupoux (2003) found that semantic and syntactic features may influence phonological processes, such as retrieving the phonological representation of the target word.

Nevertheless, differential noun-verb performances in aphasic patients could also lend support to the assumption of two separate storage mechanisms for lexemes according to their grammatical category (Caramazza & Hillis, 1991; Miceli et al., 1984; Williams & Canter, 1987) as proposed in the Independent Network Model (Caramazza & Miozzo, 1997) or alternatively, semantic and syntactic information may influence morpho-phonological processing (Bachoud-Lévi & Dupoux, 2003; Edwards, 2002; Laiacona & Caramazza, 2004). Taken together these findings of specific grammatical class impairments (verb or noun breakdown) (see Table 2) observed in both languages spoken by bilingual aphasic patients, suggest that common principles underlie the representation of words in the two languages and that common neural tissue underlies both (Green, 2008).

Neuroanatomical explanation

The bilingual anomic subjects demonstrated large variability in lesion sites (see Table 2). Verb impairments have been described in fluent aphasic/anomic patients with temporo-parietal lesions (Luzzatti et al., 2002) as well as subcortical lesions (Jonkers, 1998; Jonkers & Bastiaanse, 1996; Luzzatti et al., 2002; Tsapkini et al., 2002). Similarly, grammatical word class deficits have been reported in individuals with non-focal or diffuse brain pathology. Selective impairments for action names during picture naming have been observed in individuals with dementia (Bushell & Martin, 1997; Cappa et al., 1998; Miozzo et al., 1994; Silveri & Di Betta, 1997; White-Devine et al., 1996) dementia of the Alzheimer's type (DAT) (Cappa et al., 1998) Parkinson's Disease (PD), (Boulenger, Mechtouff, Thobois, Broussolle, Jeannerod & Nazir, 2008; Crescentini, Mondolo, Biasutti & Shallice, 2007) Alzheimer's Disease (AD), (Druks, Masterson, Kopelman, Clare, Rose & Rai, 2006). In contrast, greater impairments naming nouns (objects names) compared to (action) verbs have also been reported in individuals with dementia (Parris & Weekes, 2001), DAT (Silveri & Di Betta, Williamson et al., 1998), and PPA (Hillis, Oh, & Ken, 2004b).

The finding (i.e., verb impairments associated with 'atypical' lesions, that is, lesions outside the frontal/pre-frontal motor regions) does not support results from a number of neuroimaging studies linking verb retrieval with specific frontal lobe activation (Pulvermuller 2001; Pulvermuller et al., 1996, 1999; Shapiro et al., 2001). Instead, the finding is more in line with recent lesion and imaging research that proposes verbs and nouns (action and object knowledge) are represented within a mosaic of regions distributed over a widespread cortical network with no regional specificity for one type of word compared with another (Hadar et al., 2002; Kable et al., 2002; Luzzatti et al., 2002; Tranel et al., 2001; Tyler et al., 2001; Pulvermuller et al., 1999; Warburton et al., 1996). For verb retrieval this network can include more posterior temporo-parietal areas and/or subcortical structures in addition to frontal regions (Damasio & Tranel, 1993; Daniele et al., 1994; Luzzatti et al., 2002; Martin et al., 1995; Tranel et al., 2001).

Future Directions

The study of aphasia enables researchers to test psycholinguistic and linguistic theories about language processing and linguistic distinctions such as the grammatical distinction between verbs and nouns. Findings of neurophysiological differences in the processing of different word types (e.g. verbs and nouns) which are congruent with theoretical, linguistic distinctions are often interpreted as evidence in support of these grammatical constructs and distinctions.

This review of the literature has highlighted the fact that noun-verb differences have been exclusively studied in monolingual aphasia. Yet, still very little is known about the retrieval of different types of verbs and nouns or the factors influencing their retrieval, despite many years of research. This was demonstrated by the inconclusive findings reported in the studies described. Many factors have lead to the contradictory outcomes and include the findings that: verbs and nouns are highly variable in meaning but can also have a close relationship; lesion studies linking verb-noun dissociations with specific brain areas remain contradictory; the methodological issues and the fact that verb-noun differences have been studied in languages with different underlying forms have influenced the results.

In general, despite substantial methodological problems, the large body of evidence on verb/noun impairments in aphasia has generated a number of hypotheses to explain grammatical class effects or the functional locus of verb-noun dissociations. The lexical-semantic hypothesis assumes that verb-noun differences represent a selective loss of (word class) information at the level of the central semantic system that affects all input and output lexical modalities (Daniele et al., 1994; McCarthy & Warrington, 1985; Miceli et al., 1984). Alternatively, the lexical hypothesis (Caramazza & Hillis, 1991; Hillis & Caramazza, 1995; Miceli et al., 1984; 1988; Rapp & Caramazza, 1998) assumes that noun/verb differences arise at the level of the phonological (or orthographic) output (or input) lexicon(s) where grammatical class information is organised. Furthermore, verb retrieval deficits have led to the suggestion that the verb-noun dichotomy might be due to grammatical difficulties and/or a general syntactic disorder (Jonkers & Bastiaanse, 1998; Miceli et al., 1984; Myerson & Goodglass, 1972; Saffran et al., 1980; Zingeser & Berndt, 1990), and/or problems with morphology (Caramazza & Berndt, 1985; Tsapkini et al., 2001; 2002) issues related to verb processing. Finally, evidence from functional neuroimaging studies has revealed distinct cerebral areas correlated to noun and verb processing suggesting that nouns and verbs may be selectively damaged or spared in patients with lesions involving different cerebral areas.

So far, verb-noun processing differences in aphasic speakers of two languages are rarely reported in comparison to the large number of studies addressing the same issue in monolingual aphasic speakers. Most importantly, bilingual aphasia provides an excellent vehicle for looking at whether grammatical impairments, such as potential differences in noun and verb processing are language specific or whether they are the result of conceptual and/or linguistic differences between nouns and verbs. A further interesting aspect is whether the two languages are subserved by the same areas in the brain. If similar processing differences in noun and verb processing are observed in either language, one could conclude that nouns and verbs of both languages are processed, possibly by the same areas in the brain. In other words, neurophysiological processes involved in word processing must be primarily affected by the grammatical category of the word rather than the language in which the word is presented.

In this chapter six studies investigating verb-noun processing in bilingual aphasic speakers are reviewed. Specifically, verb-noun retrieval was described in aphasic individuals with anomia and four patterns of bilingual performance explaining verb-noun dissociations in bilingual aphasia are reported.

This finding is of major significance for theories of bilingual language processing for a number of reasons. First, the same pattern of impairment in both languages suggests that the difference is the result of conceptual and/or linguistic differences between nouns and verbs rather than an artifact of the language in question. Likewise, the same verb/noun difference in either language suggests that nouns and verbs of both languages are processed in a similar manner, possibly by the same areas in the brain reinforcing the assumption that neurophysiological processes involved in lexical access must be primarily affected by the grammatical category of the word rather than the language in which the word is presented. Second, the finding that verbs were more difficult to retrieve in languages with different underlying forms e.g in Greek (L1), a highly inflected language compared to English (L2) which is minimally inflected, supports the assumption that verbs are inherently more difficult than nouns possibly, because of more abstract differentiations in their underlying semantic/thematic or syntactic structure. Third, the finding that verbs were more difficult to retrieve than nouns in the majority of bilingual patients with anomia revealed that noun/verb differences do not correlate well with lesion site and are not exclusive to agrammatism/Broca's aphasia. Finally the overall finding that word retrieval performances were better preserved in L1 lends support to the Revised Hierarchical Model for a representational account of bilingual lexical access.

Therefore the findings make new contributions in three main areas. First, to the existing literature in relation to grammatical word class processing (verbs/nouns) specifically that for group performances. Second, to the area of bilingual aphasia as potential verb and noun processing differences in bilingual individuals were brought to light and specifically selective verb deficits were reported in both languages of most bilingual anomic patients. Third, to literature that criticizes symptom association as a poor index of functional organization in (monolingual) aphasic subjects (Berndt, Burton et al., 2002; Druks, 2002).

The overall, striking finding of greater difficulty with verb retrieval compared to noun retrieval regardless of lesion site, in a group of bilingual aphasic speakers (Kambanaros & van Steenbrugge, 2006; Poncelet et al., 2007) is of major significance. This finding represents evidence counter to the association between anomia and a reduced ability to process nouns (Daniele et al., 1994; Miceli et al., 1988; Myerson & Goodglass, 1972; Shapiro et al., 2000; Silveri & Di Betta, 1997; Zingeser & Berndt, 1988, 1990). Furthermore, the same results have been reported in studies involving monolingual anomic aphasic speakers of Dutch (Bastiaanse & Jonkers, 1998; Jonkers, 1998; Jonkers & Bastiaanse, 1996), English (Berndt et al., 1997; Caramazza & Hillis, 1995; Kohn et al., 1989; Manning & Warrington, 1996; Marshall et al., 1998; McCarthy & Warrington, 1985; Williams & Canter, 1987), French (Kremin, 1994) and Italian (Basso et al., 1990).

By and large, the bilingual findings regarding L1 and L2 noun/verb retrieval, do not seem to support the hypothesised psychological and neurophysiological distinctions between procedural/declarative memory on one hand, and anterior versus posterior (cortical) areas on the other hand. It seems that distinctions like procedural versus declarative memory systems and that between anterior and posterior language processing are unable to account for the complex cognitive and linguistic processes involved in (bilingual) language processing. However, it must stressed that this overall conclusion is based on the performances across 15 anomic aphasic bilingual subjects (Kambanaros & van Steenbrugge, 2006; Poncelet et al., 2007) on picture naming tasks in one modality only, and that the bilingual participants were not pre-selected for inclusion in these studies to support a particular theory.

Clinical Implications

The findings of the current study also have major clinical application in the following four areas: assessment, therapy, service delivery and further research.

Assessment: Speech Pathologists investigating word retrieval breakdown in bilingual aphasia have few (formal) assessment procedures to investigate noun/verb breakdown and secondly few models of bilingual cognitive processing for establishing the underlying impairment. The language tasks designed in the more recent studies investigating grammatical-category specific deficits in patients with bilingual aphasia were devised by taking into account features of both languages. For example, all verbs and/or nouns were controlled on factors known to affect their retrieval such as instrumentality, name-relation, argument and thematic structure, as well as imageabilty and word frequency in L1 and L2. It is also suggested that psycholinguistic models can be useful for establishing the underlying impairment in naming in bilingual anomia namely lemma versus word form.

Therapy: The first issue is unique to bilingual aphasia and involves the question as to which language(s) should be used in treatment. This question poses a challenge to researchers to strive for a better theoretical understanding of the various patterns of language recovery in bilingual aphasic patients, in order to develop effective treatment strategies. Given the sparse number of bilingual treatment studies and the conflicting outcomes with regards to the effects of treatment and methods more research is needed to develop theory-based treatment approaches in bilingual aphasia. Roberts (2001) has suggested that "the principles that guide unilingual treatment are also relevant to bilingual treatment" (p. 221).

The second issue is that therapy studies in (monolingual) anomia are aimed at facilitating access to the phonological word forms (and not the lemma) because the level of breakdown is assumed to be at the level of the phonological form. The findings from the bilingual aphasic studies highlight that word finding problems (even in aphasic subjects with the same diagnosis) may require different kinds of intervention based on the underlying causes/levels of breakdown. Furthermore, psycholinguistic models provide little information to develop (bilingual) treatment strategies.

Service delivery: A significant challenge to the speech pathology profession is to recruit bilingual speech pathologists with near-native proficiency in both languages. Furthermore, according to Roberts (2001) a bilingual aphasic patient takes up more of a therapist's time than a monolingual aphasic patient. For example, translating/adapting assessment tests/ treatment materials, testing and/or working in two languages in therapy or training interpreters are very time-consuming issues. Given the current economic climate speech pathologists in adult settings (hospitals, nursing homes etc) are under enormous pressure to deal with more patients for shorter durations. This will certainly have a detrimental effect on the needs of bilingual aphasic patients.

Future research: Little published information exists on language-breakdown in bilingual and multilingual individuals. Past research in bilingual aphasia has largely focused on the issue of differential performance in the two languages (see Paradis, 1995) based on descriptive case studies. However, the more recent studies investigating verb-noun breakdown in a bilingual context as reviewed in this chapter, have shifted into the area of cognitive neuropsychology and by doing so attempt to addresses a major gap in the knowledge associated with verb and noun processing in bilingual aphasia. These new studies were theoretically driven, based on hypotheses from the monolingual literature and tested on bilingual individuals. It has been argued that such studies can help further refine models of bilingual language breakdown

One reason for the lack of research in this area relates to substantial methodological difficulties facing researchers. This ambiguity may be rooted in a general lack of awareness of how bilingual participants function in varying linguistic environments. According to Grosjean (1997, 1998) many of the contradictory findings in the literature related to bilingualism could have been avoided had researchers paid closer attention to how bilingual participants were chosen. He suggests that at the heart of the problem is a lack of shared knowledge (across and within fields) as to the nature of bilingualism and as to which participant-related factors potentially affect research outcomes.

This chapter has highlighted that several factors need to be taken into consideration when choosing bilingual participants for research purposes. In order to determine the effects of bilingualism on verb-noun processing, future studies should strive to control for linguistic variables by obtaining detailed information about participants including language status, language history, language stability, language competency across domains and language demands. The patterns of bilingualism resulting from daily use and experience with two languages is highly complex and variable and there is no doubt that a bilingual individual presents a different linguistic profile than a monolingual individual.

Participant descriptions should include as many language descriptors as possible, especially those that are known to affect language performances. Lack of consideration of such information may result in inconsistent research findings across studies, which may eventually lead to a trial-and-error approach to working with bilingual clients with word retrieval impairments. At best, not reporting these descriptive variables may prevent accurate replication of research studies. Obtaining as much information as possible will improve research conceptualization, interpretation and replication. Finally, adopting a standard for describing bilingual participants will allow the field to advance theoretical knowledge of how bilingual aphasic and non-brain injured bilingual individuals process verbs and nouns in both their languages relative to other bilinguals and relative to their monolingual counterparts.

Conclusion

Future research investigating verb-noun processing in bilingual aphasia should address similar questions from the monolingual or 'mainstream' aphasia literature (Roberts, 2001) that is, combine research on current theories of verb-noun processing and current theories on bilingualism. It is recommended that researchers interested in pursuing this type of research seek more information on bilingualism before designing research projects (Baker, 2002; Grosjean, 1989, 1997, 1998).

There is no doubt that grammatical class is an important factor in the comprehension and production of individual words and this chapter highlights the need for more targeted investigations of noun-verb processing in bilingual speakers of different languages. Future studies might aim to capture different aspects by investigating the verb-noun dichotomy in languages with different underlying forms or in aphasic individuals with different types of bilingualism. Nevertheless, the growing interest in bilingual aphasia makes the study of word retrieval deficits in speakers of two (or more) languages a subject ripe for further exploration.

References

Abutalebi, J. & Green, D. W. (2007). Bilingual speech production: The neurocognition of language representation and control. *Journal of Neurolinguistics*, *20*, 242-275.

Aggujaro, S., Crepaldi, D., Pistarini, C., Taricco, M. & Luzzatti, C. (2006). Neuro-anatomical correlates of impaired retrieval of verbs and nouns: Interaction of grammatical class, imageability and actionality. *Journal of Neurolinguistics*, *19*, 175-194.

Albert, M. L. & Obler, L. K. (1978). *The bilingual brain.* New York: Academic Press.

Allport, D. A. (1985). Distributed memory, modular subsystems and dysphasia. In: S. K. Newman, & R. Epstein (Eds.), *Current perspective in dysphasia* (32-60).

Also In: M. Paradis (ed.), *Manifestations of Aphasic Symptoms in Different Languages*, (197-212). Elsevier Science: Oxford.

Altenber, E. P. & Cairns, H. S. (1983). The effects of phonotactic constraints on lexical processing in bilingual and monolingual subjects. *Journal of Verbal Learning and Verbal Behaviour*, *22*, 174-188.

American Speech and Hearing Association Multicultural Action Agenda (2000). Rockville, American Speech – Language Hearing Association.

Ardila, A. & Rosselli, M. (1994). Averbia as a Selective Naming Disorder: A Single Case Report. *Journal of Psycholinguistic Research*, *vol. 23, No 2*, 139-148.

Ardila, A. (1998). Bilingualism: A neglected and chaotic area. *Aphasiology*, *12(2)*, 131-134.

Bachoud – Levi, A. C. & Dupoux, E. (2003). An influence of syntactic and semamtic variables on word form retrieval. *Cognitive Neurpsychology*, *20(2)*, 163-188.

Baker, R. (2002). The assessment of functional communication in culturally and linguistic diverse populations. In: L. W & C. Frattali (eds.), *Neurogenic Communication Disorders*: *A functional approach* (81-100). New York: Thieme.

Basso, A. & Marangolo, P. (2000). Cognitive neuropsychological rehabilitation: The emperor's new clothes? *Neuropsychological Rehabilitation*, *10*, 219-229.

Basso, A., Razzano, C., Faglioni, P. & Zanobio, M.E. (1990). Confrontation naming, picture description and action naming in aphasic patients. *Aphasiology*, *4*, 185-195.

Bastiaanse, R. (1991). Retrieval of instrumental verbs in aphasia : an explorative study *Clinical Linguistics and Phonetics*, *5(4)*, 355-368.

Bastiaanse, R. & Jonkers, R. (1998). Verb retrieval in action naming and spontaneous speech in agrammatic and anomic aphasia. *Aphasiology*, *12*, 99-117.

Bastiaanse, R., Edwards, S. & Kiss. K. (1996). Fluent aphasia in three languages: Aspects of spontaneous speech. *Aphasiology* ,*10*, 561-575.

Bates, E., Chen, S., Tzeng, O., Li, P. & Opie, M. (1991). The noun-verb problem in Chinese. *Brain and Language*, *41*, 203-233.

Bates, E., Friederici, A. & Wulfeck, B. (1987). Grammatical Morphology in Aphasia: Evidence from three languages. *Cortex*, *23*, 545-574.

Bates, E., Wulfeck, B. & MacWhinney, B. (1991). Cross-linguistic research in aphasia: An Overview. *Brain and Language*, *41*, 123-148.

Batsiaanse, R., Bosje, M. & Fransen, M. (1996). Deficit – oriented treatment of word finding problems: another replication. *Aphasiology*, *10*, (4), 363-384.

Battle, D. E. (ed.) (1998). *Communication Disorders in Multicultural Populations* (2nd ed.). Newton, MA: Butterworth–Heinemann.

Berndt, R. S. & Haendiges, A. N. (2000). Grammatical class in Word and Sentence production : Evidence from and Aphasic patient. *Journal of Memory and Language*, *43*, 249-273.

Berndt, R. S. & Mitchum, C. C. (1997). Lexical-semantic organization: Evidence from Aphasia. *Clinical Neuroscience*, *4*, 57-63.

Berndt, R. S., Burton, M. W., Haendiges, A. N. & Mitchum, C. (2002). Production of nouns and verbs in aphasia: Effects of elicitation techniques. *Aphasiology*, *16*(1/2), 83-106.

Berndt, R. S., Haendiges, A. N. & Wozniak, M. A. (1997). Verb retrieval and sentence processing: Dissociation of an established symptom association. *Cortex*, *33*, 99-114.

Berndt, R. S., Haendiges, A. N., Burton, C. & Mitchum, C. (2002). Grammatical class and imageability in aphasic word production; their effects are independent. *Journal of Neurolinguistics, 15*, 353-371.

Berndt, R. S., Haendiges, A. N., Mitchum, C. C. & Sandson, J. (1997). Verb retrieval in aphasia: Relationship to sentence processing. *Brain and Language, vol. 56*, 107-137.

Berndt, R. S., Mitchum, C. C. & Haendiges, A. N. (1997). Verb retrieval in aphasia. 1.Characterizing Single Word Impairments. *Brain and Language, 56*, 68-106.

Best, W. (1995). A Reverse Length Effect in Dysphasic Naming: When Elephant is Easier Than Ant. *Cortex, 31*, 637-652.

Best, W. & Nickels, L. (2000). From Theory to Therapy in Aphasia: Where are we now and where to next? *Neuropsychological Rehabilitation, 10(3)*, 231-247.

Best, W., Howard, D., Bruce, C. & Gatehouse, C. (1997). Cueing the Words: A Single Case Study of Treatments for Anomia. *Neuropsychological Rehabilitation, 7(2)*, 105-141.

Bird, H., Howard, D. & Franklin, S. (2000). Why is a verb like an inanimate object ? Grammatical Category and Semantic Category Deficits. *Brain and Language, 72*, 246-309.

Boulenger, V., Mechtouff, L., Thobois, E., Broussolle, E., Jeannerod, M. & Nazir, T. A. (2008). Word processing in Parkinson's Disease is impaired for action verbs but not for concrete nouns. *Neuropsychologia, 46* (2), 743-756.

Breedin, S. D. & Martin, R. (1996). Patterns of Verb Impairment in Aphasia: An analysis of four cases. *Cognitive Neuropsychology, 13*, 51-91.

Breedin, S. D., Boronat, C. B., Saffran, E. M. & Shipley, J. E. (1999). The role of semantic complexity in verb retrieval: Part 2. *Brain and Language, 69*, 264-266.

Breedin, S. D., Martin, N. & Saffran, E. M. (1994). Category–specific semantic impairments: an infrequent occurrence. *Brain and Language, 47*, 383-386.

Breedin, S. D., Saffran, E. M. & Schwartz, M. F. (1998). Semantic factors in verb retrieval: An effect of complexity. *Brain and Language, 63*, 1-31.

Breen, K. & Warrington, E. K. (1994). A study of anomia: Evidence for a distinction between nominal and propositional language. *Cortex, 30*, 231-245.

Bushell, C. H. & Martin, A. (1997). Automatic semantic priming of nouns and verbs in patients with Alzheimer's disease. *Neuropsychologia, 35*, 1059-1067.

Buxbaum, L. & Saffran, E. (1998). Day 2: Platform Session: Semantic memory and semantic processing. *Brain and Language 65*, 73-86.

Caplan, D. & Hanna, J. (1998). Sentence production by aphasic patients in a constrained task. Brain and Language 63 (2), 184-218.

Cappa, S. F., Binetti, G., Pezzini, A., Padovani, A., Rozzini, L. & Trabucchi, M. (1998). Object and action naming in Alzheimer's disease and frontotemporal dementia. *Neurology, 50*, 351-355.

Caramazza, A. (1997). How Many levels of Processing are there in Lexical Access ?. *Cognitive Neuropsychology, 14(1), 177-208.*

Caramazza, A. & Berndt, R. S. (1985). *A multicomponent view of agrammatic Broca'a aphasia.* In: M. L. Kean (Ed.), Agrammatism New York: Academic Press.

Caramazza, A. & Hillis, A. (1991). Lexical organization of nouns and verbs in the brain. *Nature, 349*, 788-790.

Caramazza, A. & Shelton, J.R. (1998). Domain Specific knowledge systems in the brain: the animate – inanimate distinction. *Journal of Cognitive Neuroscience, 10,* 1-34.

Carlomagno, S., Blasi, V., Labruna, L. & Santoro, A. (2000). The role of communication models in assessment and therapy of language disorders in aphasic adults. *Neuropsychological Rehabilitation, 10(3),* 337-363.

Chao, L. I. & Martin, A. (2000). Representation of manipulable man–made objects in the dorsal streams. *Neuro Image, 12,* 478-484.

Chao, L. I., Haxby, J. V. & Martin, A. (1999). Attribute-based neural substrates in temporal cortex for perceiving and knowing about objects. *Nature Neuroscience, 2,* 913-919.

Chary, P. (1986). Aphasia in a multicultural society: A preliminary study. In: J. Vaid (ed.), Language Processing in Bilinguals: Psycholinguistic and Neurolinguistic Perspectives, (183-197). Hillsdale, N.J: Lawrence Earlbaum Associates.

Chee, M. W. L., Tan, E. W. L. & Thiel, T. (1999). Mandarin and English single word processing studied with functional magnetic resonance imaging. *Journal of Neuroscience, 19,* 3050-3056.

Chen, H. C. & Leung, Y. S. (1989). Patterns of lexical processing in a non native language. *Journal of Experimental Psychology : Learning, Memory and Cognition, 15,* 316-325.

Chen, S. & Bates, E. (1998). The dissociation between nouns and verbs in Broca's and Wernicke's aphasia: findings from Chinese. *Aphasiology, 12,* 5-36.

Cheng, L., Battle, D., Murdoch, B. & Martin. (2001). Educating speech-language pathologists for a multicultural world. *Folia Phoniatrica et Logopaedica, 53,* 121-126

Chomsky, N. (1981). Lectures on Government and Binding. Foris Publications: Dordrecht.

Code, C. (2000). The incidence and prevalence of aphasia following stroke. *Speakability* (Action for Dysphasic Adults), March 2.

Colombo, L. & Burani, C. (2002). The influence of age of acquisition, root frequency and context availability in processing nouns and verbs. *Brain and Language, 81,* 398-411.

Conroy, P., Sage, K. & Lambon Ralph, M. A. (2006). Towards theory-driven therapies for aphasic verb impairments: A review of current theory and practice. *Aphasiology, 20(12),* 1159-1185.

Costa, A., Miozzo, M. & Caramazza, A. (1999). Lexical selection in bilinguals: Do words in bilingual's lexicon compete for selection? *Journal of Memory and Language, 41,* 365-397.

Crescentini, C., Mondolo, F., Biasutti, E. & Shallice, T. (2007). Supervisory and Routine Processes in Noun and Verb Generation in Nondemented Patients with Parkinson's Disease. Doi:10.1016/j.neuropsychologia.2007.08.021

Cuetos, F., Aguado, G., Izura, C. & Ellis, A. W. (2002). Aphasic naming in Spanish: Predictors and errors. *Brain and Language, 82,* 344-365.

Damasio, A. R. (1990). Category-related recognition defects as a clue to the neural substrates of knowledge. *Trends in the Neurosciences, 13,* 95-98.

Damasio, A. R. & Tranel, D. (1993). Nouns and verbs are retrieved with differently distributed neural systems, *Proceedings of the National Academy of sciences of the United States of America, 90,* 4957-60.

Damasio, H., Grabowski, T. J., Tranel, D., Ponto, L. L. B., Hichwa, R. D. & Damasio, A. R. (2000). Neural correlates of naming actions and of naming spatial relations. *NeuroImage*, *13*, 1053-1064.

Damasio, H., Grabowski, T. J., Tranel, D., Hichwa, R. D. & Damasio, A. R. (1996). A neural basis for lexical retrieval. *Nature*, 499-505.

Daniele, A., Giustolisi, L., Silveri, M. C., Colosimo, C. & Gainotti, G. (1994). Evidence for a possible neuroanatomical basis for lexical processing of nouns and verbs. *Neuropsychology*, *32*, *1325-41*.

De Bleser, R. & Kauschke, C. (2002). Acquisition and loss of nouns and verbs: Parallel or divergent patterns?. *Brain and Language*, *83*, 176-178.

De Bot, K. (1992). A bilingual production model: Levelt's speaking model adapted. *Applied Linguistics*, *13*, 1-24.

De Bot, K. & Schreuder, R. (1993). Word production and the bilingual lexicon. In: R. Schreuder, & B. Weltens (eds.), *The bilingual lexicon* (pp. 191-214). Amsterdam: John Benjamins.

De Renzi, E. & Pellegrino, G. (1995). Sparing of verbs and preserved, but ineffectual reading in a patient with impaired word production. *Cortex*, *31*, 619-636.

Dehaene, S., Dupoux, E., Mehler, J Cohen, L. & Paulesu, E. (1997). Anatomical variability in the cortical representation of first and second language. *Neuroreport*, *8*, 3809-3815.

Dell, G. S. (1990). Effects of frequency and vocabulary type on phonological speech errors. *Language and Cognitive processes*, *5(4)*, 313-349.

Dell, G. S. (1986). A spreading–activation theory of retrieval in sentence production. *Psychological Review*, *93(3)*, 283-321.

Dell, G. S., Martin, N., Saffron, E. M., Schwartz, M. F. & Gagnon, D. A. (1997). Lexical Access in Aphasic and Nonaphasic Speakers. *Psychological Review*, *104(4)*, 801-838.

Deloche, G., Hannequin, D., Dordain, M., Errier, D., Pichard, B., Quint, S., Metz-Lutz, M., Kremin, H. & Ardebat, D. (1996). Picture confrontation oral naming: Performance differences between aphasics and normals. *Brain and Language*, *53*, 105-120.

Don, J. (1993). *Morphological Conversion*. Utrecht, OTS Dissertation.

Drew, R. L. & Thompson, C. K. (1999). Model–based semantic treatment for naming deficits in aphasia. *Journal of Speech, Language and Hearing Research*, *42*, 972-989.

Druks, J. (2002). Verbs and nouns–a review of the literature. *Journal of Neurolinguistics*, *15*, 289-315.

Druks, J. & Masterson, J. (2000). *An object and action naming battery*. Hove, England: Psychology Press.

Druks, J. & Shallice, T. (2000). Selective preservation of naming from description and the "restricted preverbal message." *Brain and Language*, *72*, 100-128.

Druks, J., Masterson, J., Kopelman, M., Clare, L., Rose, A. & Rai, G. (2006). Is action naming better preserved (than object naming) in Alzheimer's disease and why should we ask? *Brain and Language*, *98*, 332-340.

Edwards, S. (2002). Grammar and Fluent aphasia. In: E. Fava (ed.), *Clinical linguistics theory and applications in speech pathology and therapy*, (249-266). John Benjamins: Amsterdam/Philadelphia.

Edwards, S. & Bastiaanse, R. (1998). Diversity in the lexical and syntactic abilities of fluent aphasic speakers. *Aphasiology*, *12*, 99-117.

Fabbro, F. (1999). *The neurolinguistics of bilingualism: An introduction*. Hove: Psychology Press Ltd.

Farah, M. J. & McClelland, J. L. (1991). A computational model of semantic memory impairment: modality specificity and emergent category specificity. *Journal of Experimental Psychology: General*, *120*, 339-357.

Farah, M. J. & Wallace, M. A. (1992). Semantically-bounded anomia: Implications for the neural implementation of naming. *Neuropsychologia*, *30*, 609-621.

Ferreira, C. T., Giusiano, B. & Poncet, M. (1997). Category–specific anomia: implication of different neural networks in naming. *NeuroReport*, *8*, 1595-1602.

Ferreira, C. T., Giusiano, B., Ceccaldi, M. & Poncet, M. (1997). Optic Aphasia: Evidence of the contribution of different neural systems to object and action naming. *Cortex*, *33*, 499-513.

Ferretti, T. R., McRae, K. & Hatherell, A. (2001). Integrating verbs, situation schemas, and thematic role concepts. *Journal of Memory and Language*, *44*, 516-547.

Feyereisen, P., Van Der Borght, F. & Seron, X. (1988). The operativity effect in naming: A re-analysis. *Neuropsychologia*, *26(3)*, 401-415.

Fiez, J. A. & Tranel, D. (1997). Standardized stimuli and procedures for investigating the retrieval of lexical and conceptual knowledge for actions. *Memory and Cognition*, *25(4)*, 543-569.

Fiez, J. A., Damasio, H. & Tranel, D. (1996). Action recognition and naming impairments in subjects with left frontal lesions. *Society for Neuroscience*, *22*, 724.

Fiez, J. A., Raichle, M. E., Balota, D. A., Tallal, P. & Petersen, S. E. (1996). PET activation of posterior temporal regions during auditory word presentation and verb generation. *Cerebral Cortex*, *6*, 1-10.

Franklin, S., Howard, D. & Patterson, K. (1995). Abstract word anomia. *Cognitive Neuropsychology*, *12*, 549-566.

Gainotti, G., Silveri, M. C., Daniele, A. & Giustolisi, L. (1995). Neuroanatomical correlates of category specific semantic disorders: a critical survey. *Memory*, *3*, 247-264.

Gerhand, S. & Barry, C. (2000). When Does a Deep Dyslexic Make a Semantic Error? The Roles of Age-of-Acquisition, Concreteness, and Frequency. *Brain and Language*, *74*, 24-74.

Glaser, W. R. (1992). Picture Naming. *Cognition*, *42*, 61-105.

Glosser, G. & Donofrio, N. (2001). Differences between nouns and verbs after anterior temporal lobectomy. *Neuropsychology*, *15(1)*, 39-47

Goodglass, H. (1993). Understanding Aphasia. *Foundations of Neuropsychology*, 1-288.

Goodglass, H. (1998). Stages of lexical retrieval. *Aphasiology*, *12(4/5)*, 287-298.

Goodglass, H. & Kaplan, E. (1983). *The Assessment of Aphasia and Related Disorders*. (2nd ed.). Lea and Febiger: Philadelphia.

Goodglass, H. & Wingfield, A. (1997). *Anomia–Neuroanatomical and Cognitive Correlates* (1-221). New York: Academic Press,

Goodglass, H., Christiansen, J. A. & Gallagher, R. (1993). Comparison of morphology and syntax in free narrative and structured tests: fluent vs. nonfluent aphasics. *Cortex, 29,* 377-407.

Goodglass, H., Klein, B., Carey, P. & Jones, K. (1966). Specific semantic categories in aphasia. *Cortex, 2,* 74-89.

Gordon, B. (1997). Models of naming. In: H. Goodglass, & A. Wingfield (Eds.), *Anomia: Neuroanatomical and cognitive correlates* (31-64). New York: Academic Press.

Grafton, S. T., Fadiga, L., Arbib, M. A. & Rizzolatti, G. (1997). Premotor cortex activation during observation and naming of familiar tools. *Neuroimage, 6,* 231-236.

Green, D. W. (1986). Control, Activation, and Resource: A framework and a Model for the Control of Speech in Bilinguals. *Brain and Language, 27,* 210-223.

Green, D. W. (1993). Towards a model of L2 comprehension and production. In: R. Schreuder, & B. Weltens (Eds.), *The Bilingual Lexicon* (249-277). Philadelphia: John Benjamins.

Green, D. W. (1998). Motor control of the bilingual lexico-semantic system. *Bilingualism: Language and Cognition, 1,* 67-81.

Green, D. W. (2005). The neurocognition of recovery patterns in bilingual aphasics. In: J. F. Kroll, & A. M. B. De Groot (Eds.), *Handbook of bilingualism: Psycholinguistic perspectives* (516-530). New York: Oxford University Press.

Green, D. W. (2008). Bilingual Aphasia: Adapted Language Networks and their control. *Annual Review of Applied Linguistics,* 28, 1-23.

Green, D. W. & Abutalebi, J. (2008). Understanding the link between aphasia and language control. Journal of Neurolinguistics, 21, 558-576.

Grosjean, F. (1989). Neurolinguistic beware!. The bilingual is not two monolinguals in one person. *Brain and Language, 36,* 3 -15.

Grosjean, F. (1997a). The bilingual individual. *Interpreting: International Journal of Research and Practice in Interpreting, 2(112),* 163-187.

Grosjean, F. (1997b). Processing mixed language: Issues, findings and models. In: A. M. B. de Groot, & J. F. Kroll (Eds.), *Tutorials in bilingualism: Psycholinguistic perspectives* (225-251). Lawrence Erlbaum Associate: Mahwah, N.J.

Grosjean, F. (1998). Studying bilinguals: Methodological and conceptual issues. *Language and Cognition, 1,* 131-149.

Grossman, M. (1998). Not all words are created equal. *Neurology, 50,* 324-325

Haarmann, H. & Kolk, H. H. J. (1992). The production of grammatical morphology in Broca's and Wernicke's Aphasics: Speed and accuracy factors. *Cortex, 28,* 97-112.

Hadar, U., Palti, D. & Hendler, T. (2002). The cortical correlates of verb processing: Recent neuroimaging studies. *Brain and Language, 83,* 175-176.

Hand, L., O'Sullivan, P., Plumer, K., Gupta, J., Mackaway, K., Young, W., Costello, M., Whitty, C. & Mahananda, P. (2000). Resources for culturally diverse populations: A Sydney survey. In: *Proceedings of the 2000 Speech Pathology Australia National Conference.* Sydney.

Hart, J. Jr., Berndt, R. S. & Caramazza, A. (1985). Category–specific naming deficit following cerebral infarction. *Nature, 316,* 439-440.

Hart, J. & Gordon, B. (1992). Neural subsystems for object knowledge. *Nature, vol. 359*, 61-65.

Hermans, D., Bongaerts, T., De Bot, K. & Schreuder, R. (1998). Producing words in a foreign language: can speakers prevent interference from their first language? *Bilingualism: Language and Cognition, (3)*, 213-229.

Hernandez, A. E., Martinez, A. & Kohnert, K. (2000). In search of the language switch: An fMRI study of picture naming in Spanish-English bilinguals.*Brain and Language, 73(3)*, 421-431.

Hernandez, M., Cano, A., Costa, A., Sebastian-Galles, N., Juncadella, M. & Gascon-Bayarri, J. (2008). Grammatical category-specific deficits in bilingual aphasia. *Brain and Language*, 107 (1), 68-80.

Hernandez, M., Costa, A., Sebastian-Galles, N., Juncadella, M. & Rene, R. (2006). The organisation of nouns and verbs in bilingual speakers: A case of bilingual grammatical category-specific deficit. *Journal of Neurolinguistics, 20(4)*, 285-305.

Hillis, A. E., Oh, S. & Ken, L. (2004). Deterioration of naming nouns versus verbs in primary progressive aphasia. *Annals of Neurology, 55*, 268-275.

Hillis, A. & Caramazza, A. (1985). Representation of grammatical categories of words in the brain. *Journal of Cognitive Neuroscience, 7*, 396-407.

Hillis, A. & Caramazza, A. (1991). Category–specific naming and comprehension impairment: a double dissociation. *Brain and Language, 114*, 2081-2094.

Hillis, A. & Caramazza, A. (1991). Mechanisms for accessing lexical representations for output : Evidence from a category–specific semantic deficit. *Brain and Language, 40*, 106-144.

Hillis, A. & Caramazza, A. (1995). Representation of grammatical categories of words in the brain. *Journal of Cognitive Neuroscience, 7*, 457-458.

Hillis, A. & Caramazza, A. (1995). The compositionality of lexical semantic representations: Clues from semantic errors in object naming. *Memory, 3*, 333-358.

Hillis, A. E., Tuffiash, E. & Caramazza, A. (2002). Modality specific deterioration in oral naming of verbs. *Journal of Cognitive Neuroscience, 14*, 1099-1108.

Hillis, A. E., Tuffiash, E., Wityk, R. J. & Barker, P. B. (2002). Regions of neural dysfunction associated with impaired naming of actions and objects in acute stroke. *Cognitive Neuropsychology, 19(6)*, 523-534.

Illes, J., Francis, W. S., Desmond, J. E., Gabrieli, J. D. E., Glover, G. H., Poldrack, R., Lee, C. J. & Wagner, A. D. (1999). Convergent cortical representation of semantic processing in bilinguals. *Brain and Language, 70*, 347-363.

Isaac, K. (2002). Speech Pathology in cultural and linguistic diversity. London : Whurr Jackendoff. R. (1990). *Semantic Structures*. Cambridge, MA : MIT Press

Jensen, L.R. (2000). Canonical structure without access to verbs. *Aphasiology, 14(8)*, 827-850.

Johnson, C. J, Paivio, A. & Clark, J. M. (1996). Cognitive components of picture naming. *Psychological Bulletin, vol. 120, No. 1*, 113-139.

Jonkers, R. & Bastiaanse, R. (1996). The influence of instrumentality and transitivity on action naming in Broca's and Anomic Aphasia. *Brain and Language, 55*, 37-39.

Jonkers, R. & Bastiaanse, R. (1996). The influence of instrumentality on verb comprehension in Dutch aphasics. Paper presented at the Fifth Annual Conference of the International Clinical Phonetics and Linguistics association. Munchen, 16-18 September, 1996.

Jonkers, R. & Bastiaanse, R. (1998). How selective are selective word class deficits? Two case studies of action and object naming. *Aphasiology, voln 12, No. 3*, 245-256.

Jonkers, R. (1998). *Comprehension and production of verbs in aphasic speakers.* Unpublished PhD thesis. Rijksuniversiteit: Groningen.

Jonkers, R. & Bastiaanse, R. (2007). Action naming in anomic aphasic speakers: effects of instrumentality and name relation. *Brain and Language, 102(3)*, 262-272.

Junque, C., Vendrell, P. & Vendrell, J. (1995). Differential impairments and specific phenomena in 50 Catalan–Spanish bilingual aphasic patients. In: N. Paradis (ed.), *Aspects of Bilingual Aphasia* (177-205). New York: Elsevier.

Junque, C., Vendrell, P., Vendrell, B., Josep, M. & Tobena, A. (1989). Differential recovery in naming in bilingual aphasics. *Brain and Language, 36*, 16-22.

Kable, J. W., Lease-Spellmeyer, J. & Chatterjee, A. (2002). Neural substrates of action event knowledge. *Journal of cognitive Neuroscience, 1(5)*, 795-805.

Kambanaros, M. (2003). Naming Errors in Bilingual Aphasia: Implications for Assessment and Treatment. *Brain Impairment, 3(2)*, 156-157.

Kambanaros, M. (2007). Action naming versus verb retrieval in connected speech: Evidence from late bilingual Greek–English fluent, anomic aphasic speakers. *Brain and Language, 103, 1-2*, 73-74.

Kambanaros, M. (2008). The trouble with nouns and verbs in Greek aphasia. *Journal of Communication Disorders* 41 (1), 1-19.

Kambanaros, M. (in press). The Relationship between single-word naming and connected speech in bilingual aphasia: Evidence from bilingual Greek-English speaking individuals. *Aphasiology*. DOI:10.1080/02687030902958332

Kambanaros, M. (2009). Group effects of instrumentality and name relation on action naming in bilingual anomic aphasia. Brain and Language, 110 (1), 29-37

Kambanaros, M. & van Steenbrugge, W. (2004). Interpreters and Language Assessment: Confrontation Naming and Interpreting. *Advances in Speech-Language Pathology, 6 (4)*, 247-252.

Kambanaros, M. & van Steenbrugge, W. (2006). Noun and verb processing in Greek- English bilingual individuals with anomic aphasia and the effect of Instrumentality and Verb-noun name relation. *Brain and Language, 97*, 162-177.

Kay, J. & Ellis, A. (1987). A cognitive neuropsychological case study of Anomia. *Brain, 110*, 613-629.

Kayser, H. (1998). Outcome measurement in culturally and linguistically diverse populations. In: C. M. Frattali (ed.), *Measuring Outcomes in Speech–Language Pathology* (225-244). New York: Thieme.

Keatley, C. W., Spinks, J. A. & de Gelder, B. (1994). Asymmetrical cross-language priming effects. *Memory and Cognition, 22*, 70-84.

Kehayia, E. (1990). *Morphological impairments in agrammatic aphasia: a comparative study.* PhD Dissertation. McGill University. Montreal: Canada.

Kehayia, E., Jarema, G. & Kadzielawa, D. (1990). Cross-Linguistic Study of Morphological Errors in Aphasia: Evidence from English, Greek and Polish. In: J. L. Nespoulous, & P. Villiard (Eds.), *Morphology and Phonology in Aphasia*. New York: Springer.

Kehayia, E., Singer, F. & Jarema, G. (1996). Selective Recovery in Bilingual Aphasia: Access versus Representation. *Brain and Language*, *55*, 102-104.

Kemmerer, D. & Tranel, D. (2000). Verb retrieval in Brain-Damaged Subjects:1 Analysis of stimulus, lexical and conceptual factors. *Brain and Language*, *73*, 347-392.

Kim, K. H. S., Relkin, N. R., Lee, K. M. & Hirsch, J. (1997). Distinct cortical areas associated with native second languages. *Nature*, *388*, 171-174.

Kim, M. & Thompson, C. K. (2000). Patterns of comprehension and production of nouns and verbs in agrammatism: Implications for lexical organization. *Brain and Language*, *74*, 1-25.

Kirsner, K., Lalor, E. & Hird, K. (1993). The bilingual lexicon: Exercise, meaning and morphology. In: R. Schreuder, & B. Weltens (Eds.), *The Bilingual Lexicon* (215-248). Philadelphia: John Benjamins.

Kiss, K. (2000). Effect of verb complexity on agrammatic aphasics' sentence production. In: R. Bastiaanse, & Y. Grodzinsky (Eds.), *Grammatical Disorders in Aphasia. A neurolinguistic perspective*. London: Whurr Publishers.

Kittredge, A. K., Dell, G. S., Verkuilen, J. & Schwartz, M. F. (2007). Where is the effect of frequency in word production? Insights from aphasic picture-naming errors. *Cognitive Neuropsychology*, 1-30.

Klein, D., Zattore, R. J., Milner, B., Meyer, E. & Evans, A. C. (1994). Left putaminal activation when speaking a second language: evidence from PET. *Neuroreport*, *5*, 2295-2297.

Klein, D., Zattore, R. J., Milner, B., Meyer, E. & Evans, A. C. (1995). The neural substrates of bilingual language processing: Evidence from Positron Emission Tomography. In: M. Paradis (ed.), *Aspects of Bilingual Aphasia* (23-36). New York: Elsevier.

Kohn, S. & Goodglass, H. (1985). Picture Naming in aphasia, *Brain and Language*, *24*, 266-283.

Kohn, S., Lorch, M. & Pearson, D. (1989). Verb finding in aphasia. *Cortex*, *25*, 57-69.

Kohnert, K. J., Hernandez, A. E. & Bates, E. (1998). Bilingual performance on the Boston Naming Test: Preliminary norms in Spanish and English. *Brain and Language*, *65(3)*, 422-440.

Kremin, H. (1986). Spared Naming without Comprehension. *Journal of Neurolinguistics*, *vol. 2, No. 1*, 131-150.

Kremin, H. (1994). Selective impairments of action naming: Arguments and a case study. *Linguistiche Berichte*, *6*, 62-82.

Kremin, H. & Basso, A. (1993). Apropos the mental lexicon. In: F. J. Stachowiak, R. De Bleser, G. Deloche, R. Kaschel, H. Kremin, P. North, L. Pizzamiglio, L. Robertson, & B. Wilson (Eds.), Developments in the assessment and rehabilitation of brain-damaged patients-Perspectives from a European concerted action. Tubingen: Narr Verlag.

Kremin, H. & De Agostini, M. (1995). Impaired and preserved picture naming in two bilingual patients with brain damage. In: M. Paradis (ed.), *Aspects of Bilingual Aphasia* (101-110). New York: Elsevier.

Kremin, H., Deloche, G., Metz-Lutz, M. N., Hannequin, D., Dordain, M., Perrier, D., Cardebat, D., Ferrand, I., Larroque, C., Naud, E., Pichard, B. & Bunel, G. (1991). The Effects of Age, Educational Background and Sex on Confrontation Naming in Normals; Principles for Testing Naming Ability. *Aphasiology*, *5(6)*, 579-582.

Kroll, J. F. & Curley, J. (1988). Lexical memory in novice bilinguals: The role of concepts in retrieving second language words. In: M. Gruneberg, P. Morris, & R. Sykes (Eds.), *Practical aspects of memory* (389-395). London: Wiley.

Kroll, J. F. & de Groot, A. M. B. (1997). Lexical and conceptual memory in the bilingual: Mapping form in two languages. In: A. M. B. de Groot, & J. F. Kroll (Eds.), *Tutorials in Bilingualism: Psycholinguistic Perspectives* (169-199). Mahwah, NJ: Lawrence Erlbaum Associates.

Kroll, J. F. & Stewart, E. (1994). Category Interference in Translation and Picture Naming: Evidence for Asymmetric Connections between Bilingual Memory Representations. *Journal of Memory and Language*, *33*, 149-174.

Laiacona, M. & Capitani, E. (2001). A case of prevailing deficit of nonliving categories or a case of prevailing sparing of living categories? *Cognitive Neuropsychology*, *18(1)*, 39-70.

Laine, M. & Martin, N. (1996). Lexical retrieval deficit in Picture naming: Implications for word production models. *Brain and Language*, *53*, 283-314.

Laine, M., Kujala, P., Niemi, J. & Uusipaikka, E. (1992). On the nature of naming difficulties in aphasia. *Cortex*, *28*, 537-554.

Lalor, E. & Kirsner, K. (2001). The representation of 'false cognates' in the bilingual lexicon. *Psychonomic Bulletin and Review*, *8*, 552-559.

Lambon-Ralph. M. A., Howard, D., Nightingale, G. & Ellis, A. W. (1998). Are living and non–living category specific deficits causally linked to impaired perceptual or associative knowledge? Evidence from a category specific double dissociation. *Neurocase*, *vol. 4*, 311-338.

Laska, A. C., Hellblom, A., Murray, V., Kahan, T. & Von Arbin, M. (2001). Aphasia in acute stroke and in relation to outcome. *Journal of Internal Medicine*, *249*, 413-422.

Le Dorze, G., Nespoulous, J. L. (1989). Anomia in moderate aphasia: problems in accessing the lexical representation, *Brain and Language*, *37*, 381-400.

Levelt, W. (1989). Speaking. MIT Press: Cambridge.

Levelt, W., Schriefers, H., Vorberg, D., Meyer, A. S., Pechmann, T. & Havinga, J. (1991). The Time Course of Lexical Access in Speech Production: A Study of Picture Naming, *Psychological Review*, *vol. 98, No. 1*, 122-142.

Levelt, W. J. M., Roelofs, A. & Meyer, A. S. (1999). A theory of lexical access in speech production. *Behavioural and Brain Sciences*, *22*, 1-75

Lu, L. H., Crosson, B., Nadeau, S. E., Heilman, K. M., Gonzalez-Rothi, L. J., Raymer, A., Gilmore, R. L., Bauer, R. M. & Roper, S. N. (2002). Category–specific naming deficits for objects and actions: semantic attribute and grammatical role hypotheses, *Neuropsychologia*, *40*, 1608-1621.

Luzzatti, C., Raggi, R., Zonca, G., Pistarini, C., Contardi, A. & Pinna, G. D. (2002). Verb–Noun Double Dissociation in Aphasic Lexical Impairments: The role of word Frequency and Imageability. *Brain and Language*, *81*, 432-444.

Mackey, W. F. (1967). Bilingualism as a World Problem/Le Bilinguisme: Phenomene Mondial. Montreal: Harvest House.

Magnie, M. N., Ferreira, C. T., Giusiano, B. & Poncet, M. (1999). Category specificity in object agnosia: Preservation of sensorimotor experiences related to objects. *Neuropsychologia, 37,* 67-74.

Mandler, J. M. (1996). The Foundations of Semantic Organization. *Brain and Language, 55,* 82-84.

Manning, L. & Warrington, E. (1996). Two routes to naming: A case study. *Neuropsychologia, 34(8),* 809-817.

Marin, O. S. M., Saffran, E. M. & Schwartz, M. F. (1976). Dissociation of language in aphasia: Implication for normal function. Annals of the New York Academy of Sciences, 280, 868-884.

Marshall, J., Chiat, S., Robson, J. & Pring, T. (1995/6). Calling a salad a federation: An investigation of semantic jargon. Part 2–Verbs. *Journal Neurolinguistics, 9(4),* 251-260.

Marshall, J., Pring, T. & Chiat, S. (1998). Verb Retrieval and Sentence Production in Aphasia. *Brain and Language, 63,* 159-183.

Marshall, J., Pring, T., Chiat, S. & Robson, J. (1996). Calling a salad a federation: An investigation of semantic jargon. Part 1-Nouns. *Journal of Neurolinguistics, 9(4),* 237-250

Martin, A., Haxby, J. V., Lalonde, F. M., Wiggs, C. L. & Ungerleider, L. G. (1995). Discrete cortical regions associated with knowledge of colour and knowledge of action. *Science, vol. 270,* 102-105.

Martin, A., Wiggs, C. H., Ungerleider, L. G. & Haxby, J. V. (1996). Neural correlates of category–specific knowledge. *Nature,* 649-652.

Martin, R. C. (1986). Evidence of syntactic deficits in a fluent aphasic. *Brain and Language, 28,* 196-234.

Martin, R. C. & Blossom-Stach, C. (1986). Evidence of syntactic deficits in a fluent aphasic. *Brain and Language, 28,* 196-234.

McCall, D., Cox, D. M., Shelton, J. R. & Weinrich, M. (1997). The influence of syntactic and semantic information on picture–naming performance in aphasic patients. *Aphasiology, vol. 11, No.6,* 581-600.

McCann, C. & Edwards, S. (2002). Verb problems in fluent aphasia. *Brain and Language, 83,* 42-44.

McCarthy, R. & Warrington, E. (1985). Category specificity in an agrammatic patient: The relative impairment of verb retrieval and comprehension. *Neuropsychologia, 23,* 709-727.

McKenna, P. & Parry, R. (1994). Category Specificity in the Naming of Natural and Man-made objects: Normative Data from Adults and Children. *Neuropsychological Rehabilitation, 4(3),* 255-281.

McRae, K., Ferretti, T. R. & Amyote, L. (1997). Thematic roles as verb specific concepts. *Language and Cognitive Processes, 12,* 137-176.

Miceli, G., Silveri, C., Noncentini, U. & Caramazza, A. (1988). Patterns of disassociation in comprehension and production of nouns and verbs. *Aphasiology, 2,* 351-358.

Miceli, G., Silveri, C., Villa, G. & Caramazza, A. (1984). On the basis for the agrammatic's difficulty in producing main verbs. *Cortex*, *20(2)*, 207-220.

Miceli, G., Silveri. C., Romani. C. & Carmazza. A. (1989). Variation in the Pattern of Omissions and substitutions of grammatical morphemes in the spontaneous speech of so–called agrammatic patients. *Brain and Language*, *36*, 447-492.

Miozzo, A., Soardi. M. & Cappa, S. F. (1994). Pure anomia with spared action naming due to a left temporal lesion. *Neuropsychologia*, *32(9)*, 1101-1109.

Mitchum, C. C., Greenwald, M. L. & Berndt, R. S. (2000). Cognitive Treatments of Sentence Processing Disorders: What Have We Learned? *Neuropsychological Rehabilitation*, *10(3)*, 311-336.

Moss, H. E., De Mornay-Davies, P., Jeppeson, C., McLellan, S. & Tyler, L. K. (1998). The relationship between knowledge of nouns and verbs in a category–specific deficit for living things. *Brain and Language*, *65*, 92-95.

Myerson, R. & Goodglass, H. (1972). Transformational grammar of three agrammatic patients. *Language and Speech*, *15*, 40-50.

Nagy, W. & Gentner, D. (1990). Semantic constraints on lexical categories. *Language and Cognitive Processes*, *5*, 169-201.

Neville, H. J., Coffey, S. A., Lawson, D. S., Fischer, A., Emmorey, K. & Bellugi, U. (1997). Neural systems mediating American Sign Language: Effects of sensory experience and age of acquisition. *Brain and Language*, *57(3)*, 285-305.

Neville, H. J., Mills, D. L. & Lawson, D. S. (1992). Fractionating language: Different neural subsystems with different sensitive periods. *Cerebral Cortex*, *2*, 244-258.

Nickels, L. & Howard, D. (1995). Aphasic naming : What matters ? *Neuropsychologia*, *33*, 1281-1303.

Nickels, L. (1995). Getting it Right?. Using Aphasic Naming Errors to Evaluate Theoretical Models of Spoken Word Recognition. *Language and Cognitive Processes*, *10(1)*, 13-45.

Nickels, L. (1997). *Spoken Word Production and its Breakdown in Aphasia* (1-227). Psychology Press.

Nickels, L. & Best, W. (1996). Therapy for naming disorders (Part II): specifics, surprises and suggestions. *Aphasiology*, *10(2)*, 109-136.

Nillpour, R. (1988). Bilingual aphasia in Iran: A preliminary report. *Journal of Neurolinguistics*, *3(2)*, 185-232.

Orpwood, L. & Warrington, E. K. (1995). Word-specific impairments in naming and spelling but not reading. *Cortex*, *31*, 239-265.

Osman–Sagi, J. (1987). Action naming in Hungarian aphasic patients, *Neuroscience*, *supplement, vol. 22*, 5509.

Paradis, M. & Libben, G. (1987). *The Assessment of Bilingual Aphasia*. Hillsdale, NJ: Lawrence Erlbaum Associates.

Paradis, M. (1983). *Readings on Aphasia in Bilinguals and Polyglots*. Montreal: Didier.

Paradis, M. (1989). Bilingual and polyglot aphasia. In: F. Boller, & J. Grafman (Eds.), *Handbook of Neuropsychology*, *vol. 2* (117-140). New York: Elsevier.

Paradis, M. (1995). Aspects of Bilingual Aphasia, *Elsevier Science*, 1-233.

Paradis, M. (2000). Generalizable outcomes of bilingual aphasia research. *Folia Phoniatrica et Logopaedica*, *52*, 1-3, 54-64.

Paradis, M. (2001). *Bilingual and poyglot aphasia*. Handbook of neuropsychology (2nd ed.). Oxford: Elsevier Science.

Paradis, M. (2001). *Manifestations of aphasia symptoms in different languages*. Oxford: Pergarmo.

Paradis, M. (2004). *A neurolinguistic theory of bilingualism*. Amsterdam/Philadelphia: John Benjamins Publishing Company.

Paradis, M. (2008). *Language communication disorders in multilinguals*. In: B. Stemmer, & H. Whitaker (Eds.), *Handbook of the Neuroscience of Language*. (341-349). London: Elsevier Science/Academic Press.

Parris, B. & Weekes, B. (2001). Action Naming in Dementia. *Neurocase*, *7*, 459-471.

Pashek, G. (1998). Gestural facilitation of noun and verb retrieval in aphasia: A case study. *Brain and Language*, *65*, 177-180.

Perani, D., Cappa, S. F., Sehur, T., Tettamanti, M., Collina, S., Rosa, M. M. & Fazio, F. (1999). The neural correlates of verb and noun processing. A PET Study. *Brain*, *122*, 2337-2344.

Perani, D., Cappa, S. F., Bettinardi, F., Bressi, S., Gorno-Tempini, M., Matarrese, M. & Fazio, F. (1995). Different neural systems for the recognition of animals and man-made tools. *Neuroreport*, *6*, 1637-1641.

Perani, D., Paulesu, E., Galles, N. S., Dupoux, E., Dehaene, S., Bettinardi, V., Cappa, S. F., Fazio, F. & Mehler, J. (1998). The bilingual brain: Proficiency and age of acquisition of the second language. *Brain*, *121*, 1841-1852.

Poncelet, M., Majerus, S., Raman, I., Warinbaire, S. & Weekes, B. S. (2007). Naming actions and objects in bilingual aphasia: a multiple case study. *Brain and Language*, *103*, 158-159.

Potter, M. C., So, K., Von Eckardt, B., Feldman, L. B. (1984). Lexical and Conceptual Representation in Beginning and Proficient Bilinguals, *Journal of Verbal Learning and Verbal Behaviour*, *23*, 23-38.

Pouratian, N., Bookheimer, S. Y., et al. (2000). Optical imaging of bilingual cortical representations. *Journal of Neurosurgery*, *93(4)*, 676-681.

Pulvermüller, F. (1999). Words in the brain's language. *Behavioral and Brain Sciences*, *22*, 253-336.

Pulvermüller, F., Harle, M. & Friedhelm, H. (2001). Walking or talking? Behavioural and Neurophysiological Correlates of Action Verb Processing. *Brain and Language*, *78*, 143-168.

Pulvermüller, F., Lutzenberger, W. & Preissl, H. (1999). Nouns and verbs in the intact brain: Evidence from event–related potentials and high frequency cortical responses. *Cerebral Cortex*, *9*, 497-506.

Pulvermüller, F., Preissl, H., Lutzenberger, W. & Birbaumer, N., (1996). Brain Rhythms of Language: Nouns Versus Verbs. *European Journal of Neuroscience*, *vol. 8*, 937-941.

Rapp, B. & Caramazza, A. (1998). A Case of Selective Difficulty in Writing Verbs, *Neurocase*, *vol. 4*, 127-140.

Rapp, B. & Caramazza, A. (2002). Selective difficulties with spoken nouns and written verbs: A single case study, *Journal of Neurolinguistics*, *15*, 373-402.

Raymer, A. M., Thompson, C. K., Jacobs, B. & Le Grand, H. R. (1993). Phonological treatment of naming deficits in aphasia : model – based generalization analysis, *Aphasiology*, *7*, 27-53.

Roberts, P. (1998). Clinical research needs in bilingual aphasia. *Aphasiology*, *12*, 119- 130.

Roberts, P. (2001). Aphasia Assessment and Treatment for Bilingual and Culturally Diverse patients. In: R. Chapey (ed.), *Language Intervention Strategies in Aphasia and Related Neurogenic Communication Disorders*, (208-232). Wolters Kluwer Co. Philadelphia.

Roelofs, A. (2000). Word meanings and concepts: What do the findings from aphasia and language specificity really say? *Bilingualism: Language and Cognition*, *3*, 25-27.

Royal London College of Speech and Language Therapists. (1996). Multicultural policy.

Sacchet, C. & Humphreys, G. W. (1992). Calling a squirrel a squirrel but a canoe a wigwam: A category-specific deficit for artefactual objects and body parts. *Cognitive Neuropsychology*, *9*, 73-86.

Saffran, E. M. (1982). Neuropsychological approach to the study of language. British *Journal of Psychology*, *73*, 317-337.

Saffran, E. M. & Schwartz, M. F. (1994). Of cabbages and things: semantic memory from a neuropsychological point of view: a tutorial review. *Attention and Performance*, *15*, 507-536.

Saffran, E. M., Schwartz, M. F. & Marin, O. S. M. (1980). Evidence from aphasia: Isolating the components of a production model. In: B. Butterworth (ed.), *Language Production* (221-241). London: Academic Press.

Sasanuma, S. & Park, H. S. (1995). Patterns of language deficits in two Korean-Japanese bilingual aphasic patients: A clinical report. In: M. Paradis (ed.), *Aspects of Bilingual Aphasia* (111-123). New York: *Elsevier*.

Shapiro, K. & Caramazza, A. (2000). Grammatical class in lexical production and morphological processing: evidence from a case of fluent aphasia. *Cognitive Neuropsychology*, *17*, 665-682.

Shapiro, K. & Caramazza, A. (2001). Sometimes a noun is just a noun: Comments on Bird, Howard and Franklin (2000). *Brain and Language*, *76*, 202-212.

Shapiro, K., Shelton, J. & Caramazza, A. (2000). Grammatical Class in Lexical Production and Morphological Processing: Evidence from a case of fluent Aphasia. *Cognitive Neuropsychology*, *17(8)*, 665-682.

Shapiro, K. A., Pascual-Leone, A., Mottaghy, F. M., Gangitano, M. & Caramazza, A. (2001). Grammatical Distinctions in the Left Frontal Cortex. *Journal of Cognitive Neuroscience*, *13(6)*, 713-720.

Shelton, J. R., Fouch, F. & Caramazza, A. (1998). The selective sparing of body part knowledge: A case study. *Neurocase*, *4*, 339-351.

Silveri, M. C. & Di Betta, A. M. (1997). Noun-verb dissociations in brain-damaged patients: further evidence. *Neurocase*, *3*, 477-488.

Silveri, M. C., Perri, R. & Cappa, A. (2003) Grammatical class effects in brain-damaged patients; Functional focus of noun and verbal deficit. *Brain and Language*, *85*, 49-66.

Slobin, D. I. (1991). Aphasia in Turkish: Speech Production in Broca's and Wernicke's Patients. *Brain and Language*, *41(2)*, 149-164.

Speech Pathology Australia (1994). Speech Pathology in a Multicultural, Multilingual Society. Melbourne: AASH.

Stapleford, J. & Todd, C. (1998). Why are there so few ethnic minority speech and language therapists? *Int. J. Language and Communication Disorders*, *33*, Supplement.

Thompson, C. K., Lange, K. L., Schneider, S. L. & Shapiro, L. P. (1997). Agrammatic and non-brain-damaged subjects' verb and verb argument production. *Aphasiology*, *11*, 473-490.

Tranel, D., Adolphs, R., Damasio, H. & Damasio, A. R. (2001). A neural basis for the retrieval of words for actions. *Cognitive Neuropsychology*, *18*, 655-674.

Tranel, D., Damasio, H. & Damasio, A. R. (1997). A neural basis for the retrieval of conceptual knowledge. *Neuropsychologia*, *35*, 1319-1327.

Tranel, D., Damasio, H. & Damasio, A. R. (1997). On the neurology of naming. In: H. Goodglass, & A. Wingfield (Eds.), *Anomia: Neuroanatomical and cognitive correlates* (65-90). Academic Press: New York.

Tsapkini, K., Jarema, G. & Kehayia, E. (2002). Regularity Revisited: Evidence from lexical access of verbs and nouns in Greek. *Brain and Language*, *81*, 1-3, 103-119.

Tsapkini, K., Jarema, G. & Kehayia, E. (2001). Manifestations of morphological impairments in Greek aphasia: A case study. *Journal of Neurolinguistics*, *14*, 281-296.

Tsapkini, K., Jarema, G. & Kehayia, E. (2002). A morphological processing deficit in verbs but not in nouns: a case study in a highly inflected language. *Journal of Neurolinguistics*, *15*, 265-288

Tyler, D., Russel, R., Fadili, J. & Moss, H. E. (2001). The neural representation of nouns and verbs: PET studies. *Brain*, *124*, 1619-1634.

Ullman, M. T. (1999). Naming tools and using rules: Evidence that a frontal/basal-ganglia system underlies both motor skill knowledge and grammatical rule use. *Brain and Language*, *69*, 316-318.

Ullman, M. T. (2001). The neural basis of lexicon and grammar in first and second language: the declarative/procedural model. *Bilingualism: Language and Cognition*, *4(1)*, 105-122.

Ullman, M. T. (2005). A cognitive neuroscience perspective on second language acquisition: The declarative/procedural model. In: C. Sanz (ed.), Mind and context in adult second language acquisition: Methods, theory and practice (141-178). Washington, DC: Georgetown University Press.

Ullman, M. T., Corkin, S., Coppola, M., Hickok, G., Growdon, J. H. & Pinker, S. (1997). A Neural Dissociation within Language: Evidence that the Mental Dictionary Is Part of Declarative Memory, and that Grammatical Rules Are Processed by the Procedural System. *Cognitive Neuroscience*, 266-276.

Warburton, E., Wise, R. J., Price, C. J., Weiller, C., Hadar, U., Ramsay, S. & Frackowiak, R. S. (1996). Noun and verb retrieval by normal subjects. Studies with PET. *Brain and Language*, *119*, 159-179.

Warrington, E. K. & McCarthy, R. A. (1983). Category - specific access dysphasia. *Brain*, *106*, 859-878.

Warrington, E. K. & McCarthy, R. A. (1987). Categories of knowledge : further fractionations and an attempted integration. *Brain*, *110*, 1273-96.

Warrington, E. K. & Shallice, T. (1984). Category – specific semantic impairments. *Brain*, *107*, 829-854.

Weber-Fox, C. M. & Neville, H. J. (1996). Maturational Constraints on Functional Specializations for Language Processing: ERP and Behavioural Evidence in Bilingual Speakers. *Journal of Cognitive Neuroscience*, *8*, 231-256.

White-Devine, T., Grossman, M., Robinson, K. M., Onishi, K., Biassou, N. D. & D'Esposito, M. (1996). Verb confrontation naming and word-picture matching in Alzheimer's disease. *Neuropsychology*, *10*, 495-503.

Whitworth, A. & Sjardin, H. (1993). The bilingual person with aphasia. In: D. Lanfond, Y. Joanette, R. Ponzio, R. Degiovani, & M. T. Sarno (Eds.), *Living with Aphasia : Psychological Issues* (129-149). San Diego : Singular Publishing.

Williams, S. E. & Canter, G. J. (1987) Action-Naming Performance in Four Syndromes of Aphasia. *Brain and Language*, *32*, 124-136.

Williamson, D. J. G., Adair, J. C., Raymer, A. M. & Heilman, K. M. (1998). Object and action naming in Alzheimer's disease. *Cortex*, *34*, 601-610.

Zingeser, L. & Berndt, R. (1988). Grammatical class and context effects in a case of pure anomia: Implications for models of language production. *Cognitive Neuropsychology*, *5*, 473-516.

Zingeser, L. & Berndt, R. S. (1990). Retrieval of Nouns and Verbs in Agrammatism and Anomia. *Brain and Language*, *39*, 14-32.

Appendix 1

Variables that affect the picture naming process in individuals with aphasia.

Word frequency

During picture-naming tasks low frequency nouns (words that occur less often in the language) are harder to retrieve than high frequency nouns for subjects with aphasia (Cuetos, Aguado, Izura & Ellis, 2002; Goodglass, Theurkauf & Wingfield, 1984; Hodgson & Ellis, 1998; Howard, Patterson, Franklin, Morton & Orchard-Lisle, 1984; Kay & Ellis, 1987; Laicona, Luzzatti, Zonca, Guarnaschelli & Capitani, 2001; Zingeser & Berndt, 1988) but this is not always the case (Nickels, 1995) and a reverse frequency effect has also been reported (Marshall, Pring et al., 1998). Similarly contrasting results have been found for verb retrieval and word frequency. Some studies revealed no effects for word frequency on verb retrieval (Jonkers, 1998; Kemmerer & Tranel, 2000) while others reported a significant frequency effect (Colombo & Burani, 2002; Luzzatti et al., 2002) or an overall frequency effect affecting both verbs and nouns equally (Berndt et al., 1997).

Word Length

Subjects with aphasia are sometimes less accurate with longer words and this has been found for nouns (Colombo & Burani, 2002; Goodglass, Kaplan, Weintraub et al., 1976; Howard, Patterson, Franklin et al., 1984; Nickels, 1995; Nickels & Howard, 1995) but not verbs (Colombo & Burani, 2002). However, a reverse length effect, that is, where longer words are easier to retrieve than shorter words has also been reported in nouns (Best, 1995).

Age of Acquisition

This is (AoA), the age at which the word was first learnt has been found to equally affect verb and noun retrieval (Colombo & Burani, 2002). There is conclusive evidence that words learned early in life are retrieved faster than later acquired words in normal subjects and those with aphasia (Barry, Morrison & Ellis 1997; Ellis & Morrison 1998; Gilhooly & Gilhooly, 1979; Hodgson & Ellis 1998; Morrison, Ellis & Quinlan, 1992; Morrison & Ellis, 1995; Nickels & Howard, 1995; Vitkovitch & Tyrrell, 1995). Furthermore, it has been shown that early known words mainly nouns, may be more resistant to the effects of some forms of brain pathology than later acquired words (Ellis, Lum, & Lambon Ralph, 1996; Hirsh & Ellis, 1994; Hirsh & Funnell, 1995; Van der Borght & Seron, 1988).

Picture Complexity

In relation to *picture complexity*, the amount of visual detail/intricacy in a picture, contrasting results have also been found. Earlier studies (Sheridan, 1992; Stewart et al., 1992) reported a negative effect on noun retrieval that is, visually complex picture were harder to identify. On the other hand recent studies have found no effect for visual complexity on noun (Cuetos et al., 2002; Laiacona et al., 2001; Nickels, 1995) or verb retrieval (Cuetos et al., 2002; Kemmerer & Tranel, 2000) in picture-naming tasks for groups of aphasic subjects.

Familiarity

Familiarity refers to how common/uncommon one finds, according to their life experiences, what is depicted in the picture. Earlier studies reveal that subjects with aphasia find pictures of familiar objects e.g. "car", easier to retrieve than unfamiliar ones e.g. "hovercraft" (Funnell & Sheridan, 1992; Stewart, 1992). Other studies have found that a familiarity effect for nouns can become insignificant when other variables such as AoA are taken into account (Hirsh & Ellis, 1994; Laiacona et al., 2001; Morrison, Ellis & Quinlan, 1992; Nickels, 1995; Nickels & Howard, 1995). However recent studies support the earlier claims that object familiarity influences the accurate retrieval of noun names (Cuetos et al., 2002; Luzzatti et al., 2002) and this has also been shown for action/verb names (Kemmerer and Tranel, 2000; Luzzatti et al., 2002).

Operativity

The findings of earlier studies suggest that some subjects with aphasia are better at naming "*operative*" items that is, objects that are manipulable and experienced through more than one sensory modality e.g. a screwdriver, than those that are considered figurative" that is, harder to grasp and normally only visually experienced e.g. cloud (Gardner, 1974). Others have found that when AoA and familiarity were introduced as co-variates there was no longer a significant effect of operativity (Feyereisen, Van der Borght & Seron, 1988). However Nickels (1995) found a significant independent effect of operativity on naming performance in more than half her subjects with aphasia.

In: Aphasia: Symptoms, Diagnosis and Treatment   ISBN: 978-1-60741-288-5
Editors: G. Ibanescu, S. Pescariu   © 2009 Nova Science Publishers, Inc.

Chapter II

The Role of the Right Hemisphere in Language Processing in Aphasic Patients

Thomas Straube[*]

Department of Biological and Clinical Psychology, Friedrich-Schiller-University, Am Steiger 3 // 1, D-07743 Jena, Germany.

Abstract

The role of the right hemisphere for language processing and successful therapeutic interventions in aphasic patients is a matter of debate. New findings indicate a modulation of brain activation in right-hemispheric areas in response to language tasks in chronic non-fluent aphasic patients due to aphasia therapy. These findings show that the therapeutic intervention per se does not change brain activation across all aphasic subjects. However, therapeutic success correlates with a relative decrease of activation in right-hemispheric areas. Most importantly, initial right-hemispheric activation correlates positively with subsequent therapy-induced improvement of language functions. Thus, right-hemispheric activation prior to aphasia therapy strongly predicts therapeutic success. Furthermore, any analysis that is limited to an averaged group of patients seems to be insufficient in order to detect individual and partially opposite brain activation patterns. This chapter discusses the implication of the new findings for the understanding of neural processes involved in the recovery of language functions in aphasic subjects.

Introduction

Several studies have emphasized that the right hemisphere might be involved in language recovery in aphasic patients with left hemispheric brain lesions. Thus, by means of functional

---

[*] Corresponding author: Fax: +49 / 3641 / 9-45 142; Phone: +49 / 3641 / 9-45 154; Email: straube@biopsy.uni-jena.de

imaging methods, language-related cortical activations in aphasics have been detected not only within perilesional areas of the language-dominant left hemisphere but also within the right hemisphere at sites homotopic to left-sided fronto-temporal language areas such as the right inferior frontal gyrus and the adjacent insular cortex (IFG/IC) (e.g., Weiller et al., 1995; Ohyama et al., 1996; Zahn et al., 2004). Reactivation of perilesional areas has been suggested as being most efficient in regaining language functions (Karbe et al., 1998; Rosen et al., 2000; Heiss and Thiel, 2006). Until now, the role of the contralesional hemisphere for recovery is an unresolved issue and several, often opposite, proposals have been offered during the most recent years.

Generally, stronger activation in right hemispheric language areas has been shown in aphasics compared to healthy subjects (Belin et al., 1996; Karbe et al., 1998; Cao et al., 1999). This activation might partially be interpreted in terms of transcallosal disinhibition, an anomalous response caused by damage of left-hemispheric parts of the language processing system, and does not reflect recovery (e.g., Price and Crinion, 2005). According to this proposal, the left hemisphere normally exerts inhibitory control over the right hemisphere via callosal fibres; left hemispheric lesions would lead to an imbalance of this inhibitory control. Therefore, the resulting right hemispheric activation would not be associated with language functions. However, in some patients, right hemispheric activation was associated with improvement of language functions (e.g., Thulborn et al., 1999; Winhuisen et al., 2005), suggesting that right hemispheric activation might be related to functional recruitment of these areas for language processes. Furthermore, there is evidence that the extent of right hemispheric activation and its contribution for recovery depends on various conditions such as time since stroke onset (Hillis, 2006; Saur et al., 2006), localisation and size of the lesion (Rijntjes, 2006), severity of aphasia (Heiss et al., 1999), or time course of progression of the brain lesion in the left hemisphere (Thiel et al., 2006). In particular, patients with less severe aphasia and smaller lesions may be able to restore activation within remaining language areas or perilesional areas of the left hemisphere. Patients with more severe aphasia usually show more extensive lesions and recruit undamaged right hemispheric areas of the language processing network. The latter strategy is associated with less efficient compensation but nevertheless leads to favourable recovery in some patients (Heiss and Thiel, 2006). Thiel et al. (2006) showed that right-sided language function was found in patients with slowly but not rapidly progressive lesions and that language performance was linearly correlated with the lateralization of language-related brain activation to the left hemisphere. Thus, time might be one determining factor for a successful integration of the right hemisphere into the remaining language network in aphasic patients.

Evidence for a role of the right hemisphere in language production comes from studies that showed that a second stroke in the right hemisphere abolishes language recovery that followed a first left hemisphere stroke Some studies investigated the effects of transient "lesions", induced by repetitive transcranial magnetic stimulation (rTMS) of the overactivated right hemispheric areas, on language production in aphasic patients (Naeser et al., 2005; Winhuisen et al., 2005, 2007). Such studies allow a direct experimental test of whether or not right-hemispheric activation is necessary for language production. For example, Naeser et al. (2005) suggested that recruitment of right hemispheric areas may represent a maladaptive strategy. Thus, suppression of these areas may result in language improvement. They reported a study (Naeser et al., 2005), in which they applied one Hz rTMS to the anterior right Broca's homologue daily, for 10 days in four chronic aphasia patients. Significant improvement was observed in picture naming at two months post-rTMS, with lasting benefit at eight months in three patients. These results suggest that, in the long term, activation in the right hemisphere might be maladaptive for language recovery in aphasic patients.

However, in contrast to these findings, Winhuisen et al. (2006) showed that the right hemisphere might be involved in language functions in aphasics. Winhuisen and colleagues (2006) tested the role of activation of the right Broca's homologue in a PET/ rTMS study. In particular, it was examined whether 4 Hz rTMS stimulation over the right and left IFG would interfere with language performance in aphasic patients within two weeks after stroke. PET activations of the IFG were observed on the left (3 patients) and bilaterally (8 patients). Right IFG stimulation disturbed language production in 5 patients with right IFG activation, indicating essential language function. However, in a verbal fluency task, these patients had a lower performance than patients without right-sided TMS effect. The authors concluded that in some poststroke aphasic patients, right IFG activation seems to be essential for residual language function, although this activation seems to be less effective for language recovery than activation of the left IFG. Interestingly, in a follow up study, Winhuisen et al. (2007) reexamined these patients in the chronic phase to test whether the right IFG remained essential for language performance. PET activations of the IFG were observed on the left (two patients) and bilaterally (seven). During rTMS interference over the left IFG, all patients showed impaired language functions, indicating that the left IFG remained essential. Stimulation over the right IFG decreased language production in two patients with persisting right IFG activation. Two patients with rTMS effects over the right side in the initial study did not show these effects at follow-up. Language performance improved in all patients. Thus, as pointed out by Winhuisen et al. (2007), restoration of the left hemisphere network seems to be more effective, although in some cases, right hemisphere areas are integrated successfully in the language network. However, even if one assumes that the right hemisphere has a role for language production in aphasic patients, the question remains whether this activation reflects primary language functions or associated cognitive processes such as cognitive effort or top down control (e.g., Blasi et al., 2002; Richter et al., 2008; Raboyeau et al., 2008; see also discussion).

There is some evidence that the right hemispheric areas might be also associated with production of overlearned rhythmic word strings (Straube et al., 2008). For example, an impressive phenomenon in some patients with severe expressive aphasia is their preserved ability to sing familiar songs although they are widely unable to speak (Amaducci et al., 2002; Hebert et al., 1984; Smith, 1966; Sparks et al., 1974; Warren et al., 2003; Yamadori et al., 1977). Differential hemispheric specialisation in particular was proposed to underlie singing of familiar lyrics and intentional speaking in most right-handed subjects. While speaking would predominantly depend on the left hemisphere, singing of familiar songs would be a function of the right hemisphere (Albert, 1998; Jeffries et al., 2003; Patel, 2003; Samson and Zatorre, 1991, 1992; Smith, 1966; Sparks and Deck, 1994). This account could explain why aphasics with extended left-hemispheric lesions and a preserved right hemisphere are able to sing (e.g., Amaducci et al., 2002; Smith, 1966; Warren et al., 2003; Yamadori et al., 1977). Straube et al. (2008) investigated the role of singing during repetition of word phrases in a patient severely affected with non-fluent aphasia (G.S.) who had an almost complete lesion of the left hemisphere. G.S. showed a pronounced increase in the number of correctly reproduced words during singing as compared to speaking excerpts of familiar lyrics. This dissociation between singing and speaking was not seen for novel song lyrics, regardless of whether these were coupled with an unfamiliar, a familiar, or a spontaneously generated melody during the singing conditions. These findings propose that singing might help word phrase production in at least some cases of severe expressive aphasia. However, the association of melody and text in long-term memory seems to be responsible for this effect. The production of a melodic pattern of highly familiar and overlearned word strings seems to depend on the right hemisphere, since G.S.' left hemisphere was almost completely lesioned.

While the mechanisms associated with spontaneous recovery or the preservation of specific language functions in aphasic patients have attracted considerable research, less is known on brain processes that are associated with therapeutically induced improvement of language functions in aphasic patients. For example, functional brain imaging and electroencephalographic methods provide important tools to study the effect of therapeutic interventions on brain activation (Thompson, 2000). However, only few studies with small samples (maximum of 11 patients) were conducted so far that explored the effects of aphasia therapy or language-related training programs on brain responses in aphasics (Belin et al., 1996; Musso et al., 1999; Leger et al., 2002; Crosson et al., 2005; Abo et al., 2004; Peck et al., 2004; Pulvermuller et al., 2005; Meinzer et al., 2008). Only two studies included healthy subjects as reference for normal activation (Leger et al., 2002; Abo et al., 2004). Abo et al. (2004) investigated brain activation 7 months after aphasia treatment and found exclusively right-hemispheric activation in two completely recovered patients. In another study, individually different lateralisation shifts in frontal areas were reported in two patients after receiving intention training (Crosson et al., 2005). Peck et al. (2004) investigated times to peak (TTPs) of right-frontal hemodynamic responses as an indicator for the speed of word-finding in aphasics and found that TTPs decreased in two patients and increased in one patient after an effective two-week treatment. Furthermore, Musso et al. (1999) reported increased activation within the right superior temporal cortex that correlated with language performance after short-term therapy in four aphasics suffering from Wernicke's aphasia. In contrast, reactivation of left-frontal, perilesional areas after long-term aphasia therapy was reported in a single non-fluent aphasic patient (Leger et al., 2002). The effect of melodic intonation therapy on neural activation has been investigated in seven non-fluent aphasics with positron emission tomography revealing that left-frontal activation increased while right-hemispheric activation decreased after treatment (Belin et al., 1996). Pulvermüller et al. (2005) reported that constraint-induced aphasia therapy led to bilaterally enhanced N300 components of evoked potentials in 10 patients. Meinzer et al. (2008) investigated 11 chronic aphasia patients that recieved a short-term intensive language training to improve language functions. Overt naming performance was assessed during functional magnetic resonance imaging (fMRI) prior to and immediately after the language training. Treatment-induced changes of fMRI brain activation within the pre-training dysfunctional perilesional brain areas were highly correlated with improved naming of the trained pictures. Right hemispheric homologues showed also increased activation after therapy, but the activation was not correlated with language improvement.

Thus, the results of these studies are fairly inconsistent and it remains controversial to what extent the right hemisphere contributes to therapy-induced improvements of language functions in aphasic patients. Studies with increased sample size and with more extended analyses of correlations between brain activation and therapy outcome are strongly needed. In particular, there is a lack of studies that investigate whether brain activation in chronic aphasia may predict the success of subsequent therapeutic interventions. This analysis should be a critical test of the question whether specific activation patterns in aphasic patients are associated with prognostic trends for therapeutic outcomes.

Based on these considerations, our work group currently described an functional magnetic resonance imaging (FMRI) study (Richter et al., 2008), which aimed to investigate right-hemispheric brain function in chronic aphasic patients before and after participating in an effective treatment of language impairment. The authors measured brain activation in response to different language tasks in a final sample of 16 chronic non-fluent aphasic patients and in eight healthy control subjects. In particular, this study analysed the predictive value of brain activation for subsequent therapy outcome, and the relation between therapy outcome and therapy-induced changes in brain activation. Based on prior studies, this study focused on the most relevant region involved in recovering from non-fluent aphasia—the IFG and adjacent IC (e.g., Rosen et al., 2000; Winhuisen et al., 2005). The following paragraphs describe methods and results of this study (see also Richter et al., 2008). In the subsequent discussion, the novel data are integrated in the current models of the role of the right hemisphere in language functions in aphasic patients.

Methods

Subjects

Twenty-four patients with chronic non-fluent aphasia and eight control subjects participated in the study. Patients were recruited from several self-help groups and by public advertisement. The inclusion criteria were the following: 1) a lesion exclusively within the language-dominant left hemisphere, 2) evidence of persisting aphasia as assessed by the Aachen Aphasia Test (AAT) (Huber et al., 1984), 3) main deficits in language production but not in perception as indicated by several subtests of the AAT, 4) at least 12 months since the stroke accident, and 5) no other significant illnesses precluding participation. Eight of the 24 aphasic patients had to be excluded from further analyses. Five of these patients attended only one fMRI-session and three patients were not able to execute the tasks properly. Finally, 12 male and four female non-fluent aphasics, aged between 43 and 73 years (mean (SD) = 58.3 (9.6) years, all right handed) took part in this study. Seven patients met the classification criteria for Broca´s aphasia, seven for anomic aphasia, and two for global aphasia. Patients' characteristics are listed in Table 1.

Control subjects (four male, four female volunteers, aged between 51 and 69 years, mean (SD) = 57.6 (6.4) years, all right handed) did not report any prior head injuries, cerebral insults or language-related disorders. While control subjects were scanned once, patients were scanned directly before therapy onset (T1) and immediately after therapy (T2). There was a two-week interval between pre- and post-scans. All subjects were native German speakers and provided informed consent to participate in the study. The experimental procedure was approved by the Ethics Committee of the Friedrich Schiller University and was performed in accordance with the ethical standards laid down in the 1964 Declaration of Helsinki and its succeeding revisions.

Aphasia Treatment

Each patient participated in a two-week Constraint-Induced aphasia therapy (CIA-therapy), a behavioral treatment based on Constraint-Induced therapy (CI-therapy), developed for patients with motor deficits after stroke (Miltner et al., 1999; Taub et al., 1999). Pulvermüller and collegues were the first to show that principles of CI-therapy were also effective for the treatment of chronic aphasic patients (Pulvermüller et al., 2001). They reasoned that the demonstration that motor behavior is modifiable in patients with chronic stroke opens the possibility that another consequence of stroke, language impairment, may be sufficiently plastic also to be remedied by an appropriate modification of the CI therapy techniques used to enhance rehabilitation of movement of the extremities. When extending the CI approach to language therapy, the important question is how to implement the suited constraints in the therapeutic setting that force the patient to engage in massed practice of the relevant language functions (see also Pulvermüller et al., 2001). As in the previous study by Pulvermüller et al., the treatment in the current study intended to specifically practice language acts patients have difficulties with. One main element characterizing this method is restriction of compensatory strategies such as mimics, gesticulation, writing, drawing, and utterances that can easily be produced by aphasic patients. Therapists systematically apply the behavioral techniques of shaping as a method of operant conditioning and reinforcing strategies, i.e., the patient is rewarded for each single improvement but never criticized or blamed for any failure. Increased usage of previously neglected utterances was achieved by intense exercising during three hours per day for a total of 10 days.

Behavioral Evaluation

Aphasia diagnosis was obtained by the Aachen Aphasia Test (AAT) (Huber et al., 1984). Behavioral assessment of different aspects of language was conducted directly before (T1) and after therapy (T2). Four subtests were selected to measure language performance, including two subtests of the AAT—spontaneous speech (SS, consisting of the subtests communicative behavior, articulation/prosody, automated speech, semantic structure, phoneme structure, and syntax) and the Token Test (TT), and two subtests of the Amsterdam-Nijmegen Everyday Language Test (ANELT) (Blomert et al., 1994)—auditory (AC) and semantic comprehensibility of speech (SC).

Table 1. Patient characteristics and behavioral data.

Patient	Age	Sex	Diagnosis	SS T1	SS T2	TT T1 (reversed)	TT T2 (reversed)	AC T1	AC T2	SC T1	SC T2	BI score
A1	67	M	Anomic	3,83	4	36	38	35	40	32	40	1371
A2	60	M	Broca	3,17	3,67	12	16	45	40	43	42	476
A3	44	F	Broca	3,33	3,67	40	44	36	37	30	38	1313
A4	65	F	Anomic	4,17	4,67	50	50	47	47	44	47	845
A5	60	F	Anomic	3,83	X	50	X	40	47	40	45	1870
A6	42	M	Global	2	2,50	12	12	25	27	21	23	949
A7	62	M	Anomic	4,17	4,83	48	46	42	44	43	46	1009
A8	59	F	Broca	2,67	3,67	19	22	40	38	35	36	1160
A9	53	M	Anomic	3,83	4,5	36	23	40	45	36	33	256
A10	66	M	Anomic	4,5	4,83	50	50	45	50	44	46	1050
A11	43	M	Broca	3,33	3,83	41	44	27	29	31	43	1676
A12	60	M	Broca	3,33	3,67	31	33	30	29	27	35	1033
A13	73	M	Broca	3,17	3,67	50	49	32	37	26	38	1669
A14	51	M	Anomic	4,17	3,83	50	50	43	45	47	46	115
A15	56	M	Broca	2,67	2,67	5	7	22	24	24	29	835
A16	71	M	Global	1	1,17	10	10	35	40	32	40	617

M = male, F = female, T1 = pre therapy, T2 = post therapy, SS = spontaneous speech scale of the Aachen Aphasia Test, AC = auditory comprehensibility scale of the Aachen Aphasia Test, TT = Token Test of the Aachen Aphasia Test, SC= semantic comprehensibility scale of the Amsterdam Nijmegen Everyday Language Test, GLS1 = global score of language skills before therapy, GLS2 = global score of language skills after therapy, BI score = score of behavioral improvement; X = missing value.

As a global score for behavioral improvement (BI) the differences between test scores at T1 and T2 were z-standardised and averaged using the equation BI = ((SS_2 - SS_1) $_z$ + (TT_2 - TT_1) $_z$ + (AC_2 - AC_1) $_z$ + (SC_2 - SC_1) $_z$)/ 4. Behavioral measures were analysed using SPSS (Version 13.0, SPSS Inc., Chicago, Illinois). Patients′ scores of T1 and T2 were compared using t-tests. Effect sizes were calculated for significant effects (($M1 - M2$)/$SD1$). Statistical threshold was fixed to $p < .05$ for group comparisons.

Language Tasks

The experimental paradigm included two covert language-related activation tasks: a simple reading task (REA) and a more complex word stem completion (COM) task. Both tasks were available in two different versions, one for each time of measurement. Assignment of task version to scanning time points was balanced across subjects. Each task was performed during a separate scanning run. During the reading task participants were instructed to silently read the words presented at the screen. During the completion task the word stems had to be completed to one meaningful word silently. Each task consisted of four blocks. Between blocks a fixation cross was presented for 30 s. For the reading condition, one block consisted of 14 one- or two-syllable German nouns with a presentation time of 1.9 s per stimulus and an interstimulus interval of 0.2 s. The nouns were matched between the two versions according to word frequency and length (Ruoff, 1990). For the completion task, one block consisted of seven three-letter word stems (e.g., *han*) with a presentation time of 3.4 s per stimulus and an interstimulus interval of 0.9 s. It was assured that there were at least three meaningful completions possible for each word stem. Word stems of the two versions were matched according to word frequency of the most frequent completion in German language (Ruoff, 1990).

Pre-tests with an independent sample of aphasics were carried out to assure that non-fluent aphasics were able to solve the tasks. Based on these tests, the presentation parameters were chosen. In a final pre-test, we conducted the tasks with six non-fluent chronic aphasics and asked for comprehensibility, feasibility and speed of the tasks. Each patient reported the tasks to be adequate in speed and complexity whereas the completion task was rated as more difficult but solvable. However, to assess the task performance of patients during the scanning session, patients underwent a brief interview after completing the fMRI-session.

MRI and fMRI Data Acquisition and Analysis

In the 1.5 T magnetic resonance scanner (Magnetom Vision plus, Siemens, Medical Systems, Erlangen, Germany), two runs of 67 volumes were measured using a T2* weighted echo-planar sequence (time to echo [TE] = 60 msec, flip angle = 90°, matrix = 64 x 64, field of view [FOV] = 192 mm, scan repeat time [TR] = 4.3 msec). Each volume comprised 40 axial slices (thickness = 3 mm, no gap, in plane resolution = 3 x 3 mm) parallel to the intercommissural plane (AC-PC-plane). Additionally, a high-resolution T1-weighted anatomical volume was recorded (192 slices, TE = 5 ms, matrix = 256 x 256 mm, resolution

= 1 x 1 x 1 mm, duration = 12 min). Analysis of anatomical data confirmed exclusively left-hemispheric lesions in the patients (see Figure 1).

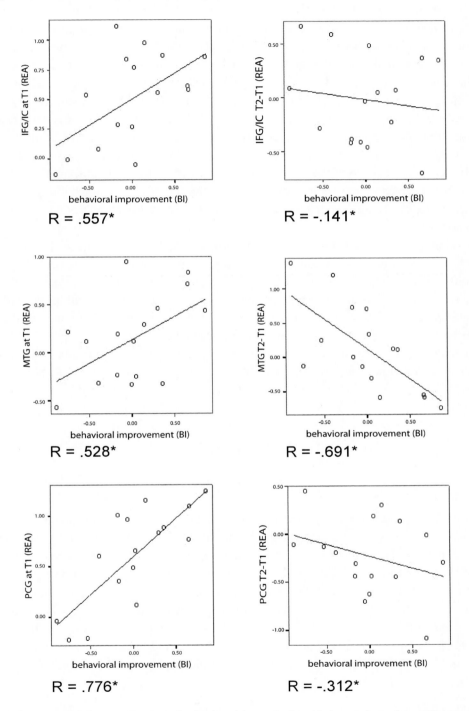

Figure 1. Brain activation in controls and aphasic subjects. Activated clusters in regions of interest at T1 in controls (x = 42, y = 22, z = 10; x = 42, y = 12, z = 8) and aphasics (x = 42, y = 22, z = 10; x = 43, y = 19, z = 31) during reading und word stem completion at the first scanning time point are shown. Statistical parametric maps are overlaid on a T1 scan. IFG/IC = inferior frontal gyrus and insular cortex.

Imaging data were pre-processed and analysed using Brain Voyager QX (Version 1.7.; Brain Innovation, Maastricht, The Netherlands). The volumes were realigned to the first volume in order to minimize effects of head movements on data analysis. The further data pre-processing comprised spatial (6 mm full-width half-maximum isotropic Gaussian kernel) as well as temporal smoothing (high pass filter: 3 cycles per run). Anatomical and functional images were co-registered and normalized to the Talairach space (Talairach and Tournoux, 1988).

Statistical analysis of fMRI-data was performed by multiple linear regression of the signal time course at each voxel. The expected blood oxygen level-dependent (BOLD) signal change for each event type (predictor) was modelled by a canonical hemodynamic response function (modified gamma function). Statistical parametric maps resulting from the whole brain, voxelwise analysis were inspected within and outside defined regions of interest (ROIs). As a consequence of the widespread lesions within the left hemisphere, we analysed only right hemispheric areas in the patient group. The IFG/IC was defined a priori as region of interest (ROI) using Talairach daemon software (http://ric.uthscsa.edu/projects/talaira chdaemon.html).

Random effect group analyses were performed for each relevant contrast: 1) activation in controls, 2) activation at T1 in aphasics, 3) comparison of aphasics and control subjects, 4) activation changes in aphasics from T1 to T2. To strike a balance between type I and type II errors, results were considered being statistically significant for clusters with peak t-values of $p < .005$ and at least 108 activated 1 x 1 x 1 mm voxels within the ROI (Straube et al., 2006; 2007). Exploratory analysis of activation in the right hemisphere outside the IFG/IC was conducted on a significance level of $p < .001$. Based on activation in the main effect analysis, additional correlation analyses between BI scores and brain activation of aphasics were performed on a significance threshold of $p < .05$.

Results

Behavioral Results

From T1 to T2 assessment, patients improved significantly regarding spontaneous speech ($t = 4.81$, $p < .001$), auditory comprehensibility ($t = 3.60$, $p < .01$) and semantic comprehensibility ($t = 2.45$, $p < .05$). Performance of language comprehension, measured by the Token Test of the AAT did not differ between time points. Behavioral data pre and post therapy are listed in Table 1. Effect sizes were calculated for significant results, showing medium sized effects for behavioral changes in spontaneous speech ($d_{SS} = .41$) and auditory comprehensibility ($d_{AC} = .51$), and a small sized effect for changes in semantic comprehensibility ($d_{SC} = .25$). Test scores before therapy did not correlate significantly with behavioral improvement score (BI), indicating that therapy-induced behavioral changes were not related to severity of aphasia.

fMRI Results

Activation at T1 in aphasics and controls

Reading. Inspection of activation in control subjects within and outside the ROI indicated a neural network involving left IFG/IC, right superior frontal gyrus, bilateral lingual gyrus, superior temporal gyrus, middle and inferior occipital gyri. Patients exhibited activation of right IFG/IC in the ROI analysis. Exploratory analysis of other right hemispheric regions in the patient group revealed activation in precentral, middle frontal, middle and superior temporal gyri, putamen, inferior to middle occipital, and lingual gyri (see Table 2, Figure 1). Compared to controls, patients showed significantly stronger activation within right IFG/IC ($t = 4.59$; $p < .005$; 940 voxels, peak voxel: $x = 42$, $y = 15$, $z = -2$).

Word stem completion. As indicated in Table 3, control subjects recruited a widespread network of activations within and outside the ROI including bilateral IFG/IC, precentral gyrus (PCG), superior temporal gyrus, precuneus, fusiform gyrus, and middle occipital gyrus, and right medial frontal gyrus and lingual gyrus. Aphasics exhibited activation of right IFG/IC in the ROI analysis (see Table 3). Exploratory analysis of other right hemispheric regions showed activation in PCG (one cluster extending from IFG/IC to PCG), middle, medial, and superior frontal gyri, lingual, middle temporal gyrus (MTG) and fusiform gyrus (see Table 3, Figure 1). During the completion task, no between-group effects were found within the ROI. Exploratory analysis showed that aphasics exhibited significantly stronger activation than controls in one cluster within the right PCG ($t = 5.26$; $p < .001$; 918 voxels; peak voxel: $x = 25$, $y = -28$, $z = 52$).

Relation between brain activation at T1 and therapy outcome

We tested whether brain activation at T1 correlated with the amount of language improvement during therapy, as indicated by BI scores. During reading, BI showed a positive correlation with activation in right IFG/IC at T1 ($r = .56$; $p < .05$; peak voxel: $x = 48$, $y = 2$, $z = 21$). Furthermore, outside the ROI, BI was positively correlated with activation in PCG ($r = .78$; $p < .01$; peak voxel: $x = 52$, $y = -11$, $z = 25$) and MTG ($r = 0.53$; $p < .05$; peak voxel: $x = 58$, $y = -46$, $z = -9$). Thus, activation of right IFG/IC, PCG, and MTG during reading predicted therapy-related behavioral outcome. Figure 2 displays the corresponding scatter plots.

For the completion task, BI was positively correlated with activation in two clusters within right IFG/IC (cluster 1 with $r = .81$, $p < .005$, peak voxel: $x = 35$, $y = 22$, $z = 11$; cluster 2 with $r = .58$, $p < .05$, peak voxel: $x = 52$, $y = 17$, $z = 2$). Thus, as in the reading task, activation in right IFG/IC predicted therapy-related behavioral outcome during word stem completion (see Figure 3).

Therapy-induced changes in brain activation

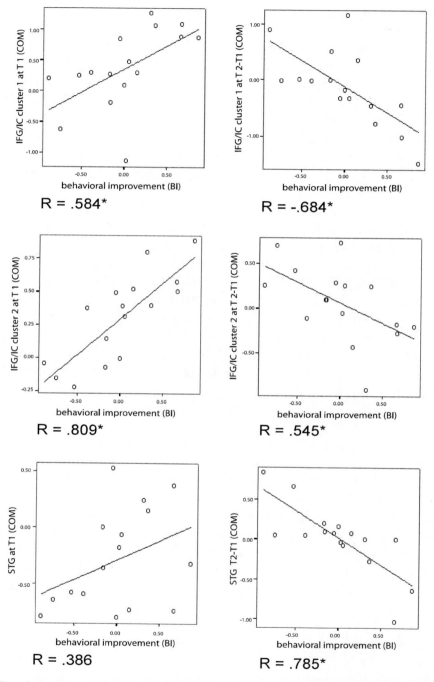

Figure 2. Correlation between brain activation and behavioral improvement (BI) during reading. Results of the correlational analyses of behavioral improvement (BI) with activation at T1 and activation change from T1 to T2 during reading (REA) are shown. IFG/IC = inferior frontal gyrus and insular cortex (x = 48, y = 2, x = 21); MTG = middle temporal gyrus (x = 58, y = -46, x = -9); PCG = precentral gyrus (x = 52, y =11, x = 25); * indicates significant correlations.

There were no statistically significant differences of activation between T1 and T2 across the whole group of aphasics. Evidently, aphasics exhibited similar activations at both time points. In the next step, we tested whether therapy-induced activation changes within the highly predictive clusters correlated with BI scores. To quantify changes in brain activation, we used the difference activation at T2 minus activation at T1. Positive correlations would indicate that a stronger increase or at least a less decrease of activation across time points is associated with more behavioral improvement. Negative correlations would indicate that a stronger decrease or at least a less increase of activation across time points is associated with more behavioral improvement.

Table 2. Activated clusters within right hemisphere in aphasics before therapy and controls during reading (REA).

Region	Aphasics					Controls				
	x	y	z	t	voxel	x	y	z	t	voxel
ROI (p < .005)										
inferior frontal gyrus/insula	49	18	23	7,75	9396	37	27	2	6,84	459
Non ROI (p < .001)										
superior temporal gyrus	49	-24	2	6,80	1809	57	-38	5	14,59	108
precentral gyrus	40	27	0	8,06	8829	38	-7	37	6,45	135
middle frontal gyrus	52	17	23	7,66	3699					
middle temporal gyrus	43	5	-42	5,87	783					
lentiform nucleus/putamen	25	-15	-4	8,61	1053					
middle/inferior occipital gyrus	31	-84	-1	19,91	29592	33	-82	-6	14,05	2403

Coordinates refer to the most significant voxel within each cluster, t = t-value of most significant voxel; voxel = number of voxels within referred activated cluster.

During reading, no significant correlation between changes in brain activation and BI was detected for the ROI analysis. However, analysis of activation within PCG and MTG indicated that activation change within the MTG was negatively correlated with BI ($r = -.69$; $p < .005$; $x = 58$, $y = -46$, $z = -9$; see Figure 2).

During the completion task, negative correlations between BI and activation change were found for the two clusters in right IFG/IC (cluster 1: $r = -.68$; $p < .005$; $x = 52$, $y = 17$, $z = 2$; cluster 2: $r = -.55$; $x = 35$, $y = 22$, $z = 11$). Figure 2 and 3 display the corresponding scatter plots for the peak voxels. Visual inspection of the scatter plots in Figure 2 and 3 revealed that activation during both tasks decreased in aphasics with higher BI scores and increased in aphasics with lower BI scores.

Table 3. Activated clusters within right hemisphere in aphasics before therapy and controls during word stem completion (COM).

Region of right hemisphere	Aphasics					Controls				
	x	y	z	t	voxel	x	y	z	t	voxel
ROI (p < .005)										
inferior frontal gyrus/insula	40	6	32	8,57	2268	49	3	20	10,23	6075
Non ROI (p < .001)										
superior temporal gyrus						52	-39	2	8,71	108
precentral gyrus	55	-12	44	6,79	1107	37	-12	59	13,72	1026
medial frontal gyrus	10	9	47	7,35	5292	4	12	47	13,28	432
middle frontal gyrus	43	18	32	9,46	5670	37	-6	44	11,59	837
lingual gyrus	13	-84	-16	7,98	12555	16	-87	-1	12,76	1620
middle/inferior occipital gyrus						34	-81	-7	10,19	1053

Coordinates refer to the most significant voxel within each cluster, t = t-value of most significant voxel; voxel = number of voxels within referred activated cluster.

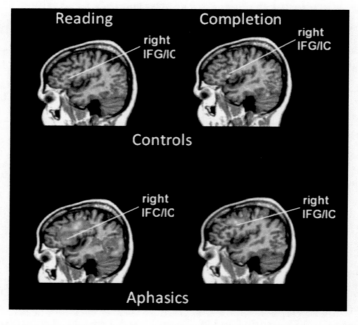

Figure 3. Correlation between brain activation and behavioral improvement (BI) during word stem completion. Correlational analyses of behavioral improvement (BI) with activation at T1 and activation change from T1 to T2 during completion (COM) are shown. IFG/IC = inferior frontal gyrus and insular cortex (cluster 1 at x = 52, y = 17, x = -2; cluster 2 at x = 35, y = 22, x = 12); * indicates significant correlations.

Discussion

The results of the study by Richter et al. (2008) provide an important contribution to the question to what extend the right hemisphere is involved in language processes. The results showed that healthy control subjects activated a distributed neural network including bilateral language related areas during reading and word stem completion. Compared to controls, aphasics activated a similar right sided network with stronger activation in right IFG/IC during reading and in right PCG during the completion task. Activation within several frontal right hemishere areas was associated with the success of the therapeutic intervention: (1) Therapeutic success correlated with a relative decrease of activation in right-hemispheric areas and (2) Initial right-hemispheric activation correlated positively with subsequent therapy success. The latter finding shows that right-hemispheric activation prior to aphasia therapy predicts therapy induced improvement of language functions.

Numerous studies demonstrated that right IFG/IC and PCG are associated with language processing in post-stroke aphasia, even though it is not resolved yet to what extent this process reflects restoration or compensation of language functions or simply artefactual activation of a disinhibited right hemisphere (Weiller et al., 1995; Cao et al., 1999; Zahn et al., 2004; Winhuisen et al., 2005; Saur et al., 2006; Price and Crinion, 2005). The finding of the study Richter et al. (2008) that control subjects activated also a bilateral language network including the classical left-hemispheric areas and the homologue regions within the right hemishere, might indicate that the language tasks used in the study of Richter et al. (2008) inherently activated language-processing regions within the right hemisphere. Involvement of the right hemisphere in language processing in healthy subjects has been also suggested by other authors (Karbe et al., 1998; Heiss et al., 1999). In an interesting study by Raboyeau et al. (2008), it was investigated whether the activation of the right inferior frontal cortex is either unique to recovering aphasic patients or present also in healthy subjects during learning of new vocabulary. Ten post-stroke aphasic patients were intensively trained to retrieve object names in French, their first language, over a four-week period. Twenty healthy subjects were similarly trained to name these items in either Spanish or English, i.e., foreign languages that they learned at school but did not master. By analogy to aphasic patients, healthy subjects had to work out the phonetic/phonologic representations of long-acquired but forgotten words. Brain activation was measured in two PET sessions before and after training. Comparable post-training performance and changes in regional cerebral blood flow including mainly the right IFG/IC were found in both groups. The authors of this study conclude, that these results suggest that enhanced activation in right-sided areas observed in recovering aphasia is not the mere consequence of damage to left-sided homologous areas, but could reflect the neural correlates of lexical learning also observed in control subjects. However, this activation in controls and aphasics might also be related to factors associated with cognitive control and effort, functions associated with right hemisphere frontal areas (see below).

Furthermore, one relevant factor for the finding of right hemisphere activation in control subjects in the Richter et al. (2008) study might be also associated with age of subjects, since rather aged subjects were investigated. It is known that age of subjects per se affects lateralization of brain activation during language and other cognitive tasks (e.g., Rajah and

Esposito, 2005; Szaflarski et al., 2006). Generally, the left-lateralized brain activation during language tasks decreases with increasing age of subjects (Szaflarski et al., 2006). This effect might be also related to factors such as increased cognitive control and effort in the elderly during language tasks.

The most important finding of the study of Richter et al. is that activation within the right hemisphere predicts therapy success and that changes in brain activation across scanning sessions correlate with the behavioral data. As described in the introduction, right hemispheric activation in aphasics has mainly been suggested to signal an inferior strategy (Karbe et al., 1999; Rosen et al., 2000; Heiss and Thiel, 2006). This might implicate that subjects with stronger right-lateralized activation might benefit more from intense language training resulting in more efficient strategies of language processing. A critical test of the question whether right-hemispheric activation is associated with good or bad prognoses of further improvement in language functions following therapeutic interventions is the investigation of the relation between pre-therapy activation and therapy outcome. Effectively, Richter et al. found positive correlations between activation of frontal language related areas (IFG/IC and PCG) and BI scores in the aphasic group indicating that brain activation prior to treatment can predicted therapeutic success of chronic, non-fluent aphasics. These findings suggest that, even if stronger activation of right language related areas reflects an inferior strategy of recovery in the chronic state, this strategy seems to be associated with better improvement after subsequent interventions. Thus, this effect might be based on a greater potential for further improvement if the current reorganization strategy was suboptimal.

The different patterns of activation and the resulting positive correlation might be associated with differences in cognitive effort while solving the reading and completion tasks. A relation between effort and activation would be in line with previous findings showing an association between the amount of neural activation in the right hemisphere and the computational demands of the language task (e.g., Just et al., 1996) and with suggestions by several authors (see below). Thus, aphasics with more effort might be those patients who experience more difficulties with the tasks. They might also be those patients who show more sedulity during training and therefore benefit most according to language improvement. Thus, individual differences in motivation and effort might influence both—extent of brain activation and therapy outcome.

Remarkably, the study of Richter et al. did not find activation changes from T1 to T2 across the whole group of 16 aphasics due to CI-aphasia therapy. Thus, there was no therapy induced up or down regulation of activation in right frontal areas. Nevertheless, suggesting that a lack of therapy-induced activation changes may also be a result of individual differences in behavioral improvement, the authors investigated correlations between language improvement and activation changes. In line with this hypothesis, negative correlations between BI and activation changes in right IFG/IC and MTG were detected, suggesting that patients indeed show different reorganisation strategies depending on therapy outcome. Activation within the right IFG/IC represents a compensatory strategy due to the loss of left-frontal classical language processing areas. The MTG has previously been reported to be activated bilaterally during retrieval of phonological and semantic codes during word reading (Hagoort et al., 1999). Visual inspection of the scatter plots showed that activation in these areas decreased in aphasics with higher BI scores and increased in aphasics with lower BI scores. Thus, the negative correlation did not simply reflect a stronger decrease of activation in patients with better therapeutic outcomes. The reduction of right hemispheric activation in aphasics characterised by high improvement might indicate a new strategy of language processing. As a result of sufficient improvements of language functions, less effort might be required at T2 compared to T1 to solve the language tasks. In contrast, patients with poor improvement may attempt to put more effort in using additional strategies after therapy but fail to restore more efficient language capacities. This is reflected by increased activation in those patients.

Saur et al. (2006) also suggested that up regulation of right-hemispheric areas in aphasic patients depends on the level of relative task difficulty and involvement of complementary cognitive effort. In their study, Saur et al. (2006) aimed to identify the dynamics of reorganization in the language system in aphasic patients by repeated fMRI examinations with parallel language testing from the acute to the chronic stage. All patients recovered clinically as shown by a several aphasia tests. In the acute phase, patient showed little activation of non-infarcted left-hemispheric language structures, while in the subacute phase a large increase of activation in the bilateral language network with peak activation in the right Broca-homologue was observed. Furthermore, this activation correlated with improved language function. In the chronic phase, a normalization of activation with a re-shift of peak activation to left-hemispheric language areas was observed, associated with further language improvement. According to the authors, the data suggest that brain reorganization during language recovery may proceed in at least three phases. First, there is strongly reduced activation of remaining left language areas in the acute phase. This might be associated with general reduction in language activation and low demand for cognitively controlling language performance. In the intermediate stage of recovery, there is an upregulation of brain activation with recruitment of homologue language zones, which correlates with language improvement. In this stage, the language areas are partially recovering but are working at a suboptimal level. Thus, there is a strong requirement for cognitive effort and control, which is associated with strong activation in the right inferior frontal regions. In the last—the chronic—stage, a normalization of activation with predominantly activation in the left hemisphere is observed. Given that language performance has continuously increased, this pattern might indicate a decreased need for additional control from right IFG/IC.

A transient role of the right hemisphere for learning and top-down control of language processing has been proposed also by Blasi et al. (2002). Blasi et al. showed that patients with left frontal lesions and partially recovered aphasia learn, at a normal rate, a novel word retrieval task that requires the damaged cortex. Verbal learning was accompanied by specific response decrements in right frontal and right occipital cortex, strongly supporting the compensatory role of the right hemisphere.

In summary, considering the latter studies and the data of Richter et al. (2008), a compensatory role of the right hemisphere in language production is the most likely explanation for right hemisphere brain activation in aphasic patients. In particular, the findings of Richter et al. (2008) suggest that aphasics exhibit stronger activations in right language-related areas probably as a result of less effective strategies for language processing and increased compensatory effort. Most importantly, activation of language-relevant right hemispheric regions before therapy is highly predictive for therapy outcome. After therapy, activation of these regions decreases in aphasics with high behavioural improvements, and partially increases in aphasics with lower behavioral improvements. This seems to indicate that, depending on compensatory strategies prior to the therapy, different therapy outcomes in both brain activation and behavioural improvement can be expected. As a result of sufficient improvements in language functions, less effort might be required to solve the language tasks after the therapy in those patients with high therapy success (but partially suboptimal recovery processes before therapy). In contrast, patients with poor improvement may attempt to put more effort into using additional strategies after therapy but fail to restore more efficient language capacities. This is reflected by increased activation in right-hemispheric areas in those patients. The results of Richter et al. provide the first evidence that right hemispheric brain activation before and after therapeutic intervention is associated with individual differences in language improvement in chronic aphasia. They suggest that any analysis that is limited to the average group data seems to be insufficient in order to detect these individual and partially opposite brain activation patterns.

References

Abo, M; Senoo, A; Watanabe, S; Miyano, S; Doseki, K; Sasaki, N; et al. Language-related brain function during word repetition in post-stroke aphasics. *Neuroreport*, 2004, 15, 1891-1894.

Albert, M; Sparks, RW; Helm, NA. Melodic intonation therapy for aphasia. *Archives of Neurology*, 1973, 29, 130-131.

Albert, M. (1998). Treatment of aphasia. *Archives of Neurology*, 55(11), 1417-1419.

Amaducci, L; Grassi, E; Boller, F. Maurice Ravel and right hemisphere musical creativity: Influence of disease on his last musical works? *European Journal of Neurology*, 2002, 9, 75-82.

Belin, P; VanEeckhout, P; Zilbovicius, M; Remy, P; Francois, C; Guillaume, S; et al. Recovery from nonfluent aphasia after melodic intonation therapy: A PET study. *Neurology*, 1996, 47, 1504-1511.

Blasi, V; Young, AC; Tansy, AP; Petersen, SE; Snyder, AZ; Corbetta, M. Word retrieval learning modulates right frontal cortex in patients with left frontal damage. *Neuron*, 2002, 36(1), 159-70.

Blomert, L; Kean, ML; Koster, C; Schokker, J. Amsterdam-Nijmegen Everyday Language Test - Construction, Reliability and Validity. *Aphasiology*, 1994, 8, 381-407.

Cao, Y; Vikingstad, EM; George, KP; Johnson, AF; Welch, KMA. Cortical language activation in stroke patients recovering from aphasia with functional MRI. *Stroke*, 1999, 30, 2331-2340.

Crosson, B; Moore, AB; Gopinath, K; White, KD; Wierenga, CE; Gaiefsky, ME; et al. Role of the right and left hemispheres in recovery of function during treatment of intention in aphasia. *Journal of Cognitive Neuroscience*, 2005, 17, 392-406.

Hagoort, P; Indefrey, P; Brown, C; Herzog, H; Steinmetz, H; Seitz, RJ. The neural circuitry involved in the reading of German words and pseudowords: A PET study. *Journal of Cognitive Neuroscience*, 1999, 11, 383-398.

Heiss, WD; Kessler, J; Thiel, A; Ghaemi, M; Karbe, H. Differential capacity of left and right hemispheric areas for compensation of poststroke aphasia. *Annals of Neurology*, 1999, 45, 430-438.

Heiss, WD; Thiel, A. A proposed regional hierarchy in recovery of post-stroke aphasia. *Brain and Language*, 2006, 98, 118-123.

Hillis, AE. The right place at the right time? *Brain*, 2006, 129, 1351-1353.

Huber, W; Poeck, K; Willmes, K. The Aachen Aphasia Test. *Adv Neurol.*, 1984, 42, 291-303.

Just, MA; Carpenter, PA; Keller, TA; Eddy, WF; Thulborn, KR. Brain activation modulated by sentence comprehension. *Science*, 1996, 274, 114-116.

Karbe, H; Thiel, A; Weber-Luxenburger, G; Herholz, K; Kessler, J; Heiss, WD. Brain plasticity in poststroke aphasia: What is the contribution of the right hemisphere? *Brain and Language*, 1998, 64, 215-230.

Leger, A; Demonet, JF; Ruff, S; Aithamon, B; Touyeras, B; Puel, M; et al. Neural substrates of spoken language rehabilitation in an aphasic patient: An fMRI study. *Neuroimage*, 2002, 17, 174-183.

Meinzer, M; Flaisch, T; Breitenstein, C; Wienbruch, C; Elbert, T; Rockstroh, B. Functional re-recruitment of dysfunctional brain areas predicts language recovery in chronic aphasia. *Neuroimage*, 2008 Feb 15, 39(4), 2038-46. Epub 2007 Oct 18.

Miltner, WHR; Bauder, H; Sommer, M; Taub, E. Constraint-induced movement therapy—Results of a behavioral psychology training program for motor rehabilitation of stroke patients. *Verhaltenstherapie*, 1999, 9, 50-50.

Musso, M; Weiller, C; Kiebel, S; Muller, SP; Bulau, P; Rijntjes, M. Training-induced brain plasticity in aphasia. *Brain*, 1999, 122, 1781-1790.

Naeser, MA; Martin, PI; Baker, EH; Hodge, SM; Sczerzenie, SE; Nicholas, M; et al. Overt propositional speech in chronic nonfluent aphasia studied with the dynamic susceptibility contrast fMRI method. *Neuroimage*, 2004, 22, 29-41.

Ohyama, M; Senda, M; Kitamura, S; Ishii, K; Mishina, M; Terashi, A. Role of the nondominant hemisphere and undamaged area during word repetition in poststroke aphasics - A PET activation study. *Stroke*, 1996, 27, 897-903.

Peck, KK; Moore, AB; Crosson, BA; Gaiefsky, M; Gopinath, KS; White, K; et al. Functional magnetic resonance imaging before and after aphasia therapy—Shifts in hemodynamic time to peak during an overt language task. *Stroke*, 2004, 35, 554-559.

Pedersen, PM; Jorgensen, HS; Nakayama, H; Raaschou, HO; Olsen, TS. Aphasia in Acute Stroke - Incidence, Determinants, and Recovery. *Annals of Neurology*, 1995, 38, 659-666.

Price, CJ; Crinion, J. The latest on functional imaging studies of aphasic stroke. *Current Opinion in Neurology*, 2005, 18, 429-434.

Pulvermuller, F; Hauk, O; Zohsel, K; Neininger, B; Mohr, B. Therapy-related reorganization of language in both hemispheres of patients with chronic aphasia. *Neuroimage*, 2005, 28, 481-489.

Pulvermuller, F; Neininger, B; Elbert, T; Mohr, B; Rockstroh, B; Koebbel, P; et al. Constraint-induced therapy of chronic aphasia after stroke. *Stroke*, 2001, 32, 1621-1626.

Raboyeau, G; De Boissezon, X; Marie, N; Balduyck, S; Puel, M; Bézy, C; Démonet, JF; Cardebat, D. Right hemisphere activation in recovery from aphasia: lesion effect or function recruitment? *Neurology*, 2008 Jan 22, 70(4), 290-8.

Rajah, MN; D'Esposito, M. Region-specific changes in prefrontal function with age: a review of PET and fMRI studies on working and episodic memory. *Brain*, 2006, 128(Pt 9), 1964-83.

Richter, M; Miltner, WH; Straube, T. Association between therapy outcome and right-hemispheric activation in chronic aphasia. *Brain*, 2008, 131(Pt 5), 1391-401.

Rijntjes, M. Mechanisms of recovery in stroke patients with hemiparesis or aphasia: new insights, old questions and the meaning of therapies. *Current Opinion in Neurology*, 2006, 19, 76-83.

Rosen, HJ; Petersen, SE; Linenweber, MR; Snyder, AZ; White, DA; Chapman, L; et al. Neural correlates of recovery from aphasia after damage to left inferior frontal cortex. *Neurology*, 2000, 55, 1883-1894.

Ruoff, A; editor. *Häufigkeitswörterbuch gesprochener Sprache. Gesondert nach Wortarten: alphabetisch, rückläufig-alphabetisch und nach Häufigkeit geordnet.* Tuebingen, Germany: Niemeyer, 1990.

Saur, D; Lange, R; Baumgaertner, A; Schraknepper, V; Willmes, K; Rijntjes, M; et al. Dynamics of language reorganization after stroke. *Brain*, 2006, 129, 1371-1384.

Straube, T; Glauer, M; Dilger, S; Mentzel, HJ; Miltner, WHR. Effects of cognitive-behavioral therapy on brain activation in specific phobia. *Neuroimage*, 2006, 29, 125-135.

Straube, T; Schulz, A; Geipel, K; Mentzel, HJ; Miltner, WH. Dissociation between singing and speaking in expressive aphasia: the role of song familiarity. *Neuropsychologia*, 2008, 46(5), 1505-12.

Straube, T; Weiss, T; Mentzel, HJ; Miltner, WHR. Time course of amygdala activation during aversive conditioning depends on attention. *Neuroimage*, 2007, 34, 462-469.

Szaflarski, JP; Holland, SK; Schmithorst, VJ; Byars, AW. fMRI study of language lateralization in children and adults. *Hum Brain Mapp.*, 2006, 27(3), 202-12.

Talairach, P; Tournoux, J; editors. *A Stereotactic Coplanar Atlas of the Human Brain.* Stuttgart, Germany: Thieme, 1988.

Taub, E; Uswatte, G; Pidikiti, R. Constraint-Induced Movement Therapy: A new family of techniques with broad application to physical rehabilitation - A clinical review. *Journal of Rehabilitation Research and Development*, 1999, 36, 237-251.

Thompson, CK. The neurobiology of language recovery in aphasia. *Brain and Language*, 2000, 71, 245-248.

Thulborn, KR; Carpenter, PA; Just, MA. Plasticity of language-related brain function during recovery from stroke. *Stroke*, 1999, 30, 749-754.

Wade, DT; Hewer, RL; David, RM; Enderby, PM. Aphasia after Stroke - Natural-History and Associated Deficits. *Journal of Neurology Neurosurgery and Psychiatry*, 1986, 49, 11-16.

Warren, JD; Warren, JE; Fox, NC; Warrington, EK. (2003). Nothing to say, something to sing: primary progressive dynamic aphasia. *Neurocase*, 9, 140-155.

Weiller, C; Isensee, C; Rijntjes, M; Huber, W; Muller, S; Bier, D; et al. Recovery from Wernickes Aphasia - a Positron Emission Tomographic Study. *Annals of Neurology*, 1995, 37, 723-732.

Winhuisen, L; Thiel, A; Schumacher, B; Kessler, J; Rudolf, J; Haupt, WF; et al. Role of the contralateral inferior frontal gyrus in recovery of language function in poststroke aphasia - A combined repetitive transcranial magnetic stimulation and positron emission tomography study. *Stroke*, 2005, 36, 1759-1763.

Yamadori, A; Osumi, Y; Masuhara, S; Okubo, M. (1977). Preservation of singing in Broca's aphasia. *Journal of neurology, neurosurgery, and psychiatry*, 40, 221-224.

Zahn, R; Drews, E; Specht, K; Kemeny, S; Reith, W; Willmes, K; et al. Recovery of semantic word processing in global aphasia: a functional MRI study. *Cognitive Brain Research*, 2004, 18, 322-336.

In: Aphasia: Symptoms, Diagnosis and Treatment
Editors: G. Ibanescu, S. Pescariu

ISBN: 978-1-60741-288-5
© 2009 Nova Science Publishers, Inc.

Chapter III

Category and Letter Fluency in Primary Progressive Aphasia, Semantic Dementia, and Alzheimer's Disease

Cecile A. Marczinski[*]
Northern Kentucky University, USA

Abstract

Many patients with different degenerative dementias also exhibit aphasia in varying degrees. Recent evidence has suggested that the fluency test might be a powerful assessment to aid in diagnostic decisions of dementia and could be deemed the one-minute mental status examination. Verbal fluency tasks consist of generating words from a semantic category (e.g., animals) or words beginning with a given letter (e.g., the letter 'S') within a specified time limit, such as 60 seconds. The use of the fluency task as a quick mental status exam is not only appealing in its brevity to administer but also in the potential richness of the data acquired. The present chapter presents findings from a study that compared how patients with different degenerative dementia syndromes with aphasia performed on category and letter fluency tasks. Patients with primary progressive aphasia, semantic dementia, and Alzheimer's disease were compared with normal controls on fluency tasks as these three disease conditions are often difficult to distinguish from one another using general cognitive screens and neuroimaging, particularly at the early stages of disease onset. The results from this study comparing these patients with aphasia reveal that category and letter fluency tasks may be more helpful in distinguishing various dementia syndromes from normal controls and from one another than the more general cognitive screens that are typically used to assess dementia. In summary, this chapter expands and improves upon the currently accepted methodology used in the diagnosis of dementia, particularly when aphasia is a core symptom.

[*] Corresponding author: Department of Psychology, Northern Kentucky University, 349 BEP, 1 Nunn Drive, Highland Heights, KY, 41099, P. (859) 572-1438, F. (859) 572-6085, E. marczinskc1@nku.edu

Background

Aphasia is the loss of the ability to produce and/or comprehend language, due to injury or damage to brain areas specialized for these functions. The patient may exhibit a variety of language difficulties including: being unable to comprehend language, being unable to pronounce words, being unable to name objects, being unable to speak spontaneously, being unable to repeat phrases or persistently repeating phrases (Kertesz, 1979). Historically, the awareness that a brain injury can impair speech has existed since ancient times. The oldest recorded documentation is in an Egyptian papyrus from approximately 1600 B.C. In this surgical papyrus, guidelines are provided for how to treat victims of battle, depending on the symptoms and injuries. Two cases of head wounds to the temple are described with the associated loss of speech (Roth & Heilman, 2000). Despite the fact that the awareness of aphasia may have a long history, practitioners still struggle with the appropriate methods to diagnose diseases with aphasia as a symptom, even today.

Aphasia can occur suddenly, such as with a traumatic brain injury or stroke. A patient may be speak eloquently one minute, and then suddenly be unable to name a pencil when the object is presented to him or her, such as when suffering from a stroke. However, aphasia can also develop slowly over time, such as with certain progressive neurological diseases, such as Alzheimer's disease, primary progressive aphasia, and semantic dementia. Arnold Pick was the first to report of a patient with progressive aphasia (a progressive loss of the ability to produce and/or comprehend language indicating a disease process is present) and this report was the basis of the concept of Pick's disease (Pick, 1892). In his report, he described the aphasia as being caused by a single circumscribed atrophic process in the brain and he established the concept of focal atrophy causing a specific behavioral syndrome. There are a variety of disease conditions that cause slowly developing aphasia.

Distinguishing between the different dementia syndromes with aphasia is a common diagnostic dilemma facing the clinician assessing a patient presenting with symptoms of a dementia syndrome (Feldman & Kertesz, 2001; Pasquier, 1999). In an older person, family members are always more vigilant about memory impairment since the general public is familiar with Alzheimer's disease (AD). One of the most common causes of dementia (Andreasen et al., 1999; Ostbye et al., 2008), AD has memory impairment as one of its defining features. As such, memory impairment is often synonymous with dementia in the general public. Routinely forgetting where one parked his car or forgetting to turn off the stove may be observations that lead family members to request assessment of their relative for dementia. However, family members may also notice problems with language. Increased difficulty in finding words, saying the inappropriate word, or omitting words may a sign that something in the brain is going progressively wrong. These language problems can be common in AD (Appell et al., 1982) but may also indicate other neurological degenerative conditions.

While many dementia patients are initially brought to the attention of physicians because of memory problems, there is also a significant group of dementia patients that have language problems as the primary complaint. A growing body of research is establishing that nearly one quarter of degenerative dementias, particularly those with a presenile onset (before age 65), can be caused by diseases variously termed Pick disease (Pick, 1892), frontotemporal dementia (Gustafson, 1987; Neary et al., 1986), primary progressive aphasia (Mesulam, 1987), and semantic dementia (Hodges et al., 1992). These syndromes do not have episodic memory impairment as a primary feature (although memory problems can be secondary), but do seem to have considerable overlap with each other and aphasia is a common symptom (Kertesz, 2001). Since these syndromes often present in late middle age, there is often a misperception that the patient is still too young to be diagnosed with dementia. An additional challenge for diagnosis is that the characteristic features of language difficulties are less likely to be considered as part of the dementia spectrum, resulting in delays in identification of a problem or misdiagnosis. Further difficulty in distinguishing these various dementias from one another and from AD is caused by the problem that general cognitive screens and neuroimaging are not particularly helpful in diagnosis at the early stages of disease onset (Heidler-Gary et al., 2007; Perry & Hodges, 2000). The overlap in clinical profiles of the degenerative dementias, particularly as dementia progresses, makes clinical differential diagnosis a challenge (Jobst et al., 1997). Specific neurological tests have been developed to test for aphasia for these syndromes, such as the Western Aphasia Battery (Kertesz, 2006; Kertesz & Poole, 2004; Shewan & Kertesz, 1980). Many physicians rely on these traditional approaches at differential diagnosis. However, these tests take a long time to administer and it has been suggested that a new and different approach using brief tests is warranted (Blair et al., 2006; Wichlund et al., 2004).

Epidemiology of Aphasia in Dementia

Accurate prevalence estimates of dementia and aphasia in dementia are important for public health, long-term care planning, and cost-perspectives. Many estimates of prevalence of dementia have been made, but the exact rates are unknown, especially for dementia with aphasia. Studies have estimated prevalence rates of dementia using data from regional epidemiological studies, billing records, and death certificates with varying results. For example, Ostbye et al. (2008) estimated the proportion of seniors with dementia from three independent data sources in the United States. Estimates of dementia occurrence ranged from 6.3% of all seniors (when estimated from death certificates) to 13.0% (when estimated from Medicare claims). There is general agreement that AD is the most common form of dementia, accounting for approximately 1/3 of cases (Andreasen et al., 1999; Ostbye et al., 2008). Also, the prevalence of dementia is rising while risk factors for dementia, such as stroke, are declining (Ayyagari et al., 2007; Ostbye et al., 2008).

There are several reasons why there are variable prevalence estimates of various dementia syndromes. First, different diagnostic systems are used (e.g., ICD-9, DMI-IV, CERAD) (Ostbye et al., 2008). Second, many studies only examine participants ages 65 and older, while some dementias begin before that, particular for the dementias with aphasia as the primary concern. Third, there are inconsistencies in terminology in the literature. For example, it has been suggested that Primary Progressive Aphasia is the left-hemisphere variant of Frontotemporal Dementia (Neary et al., 1993; Snowden & Neary, 1993), leading to some cases of Primary Progressive Aphasia in the literature being referred to as Frontotemporal Dementia, meaning a language disorder form of Frontotemporal Dementia and not the disinhibition disorder. However, despite confusion over terminology, it is clear that the group of dementia syndromes without episodic memory loss as the primary feature contribute to a large proportion of patients presenting with dementia. Approximately 20% to 40% of dementia is caused by diseases other than Alzheimer's disease, including dementia associated with cerebrovascular disease, dementia associated with extrapyramidal features, and the frontotemporal dementias (which encompass the progressive aphasias) (Knopman, 2001). It has been reported that up to 20% of cases of degenerative dementias on autopsy are due to frontotemporal dementia alone (Heston & Mastri, 1982; Gustafson, 1993). Furthermore, the changing age structure of the U.S. population will markedly affect the future incidence and prevalence of all dementia syndromes, including those with aphasia as a symptom. Prevalence estimates of Alzheimer's disease using 2000 census data indicated that there were 4.5 million persons with AD in the U.S. population. By 2050, this number is estimated to triple to 13.2 million (Hebert et al., 2003).

Thus far, there has been a paucity of research on the epidemiology of non-AD dementias, so the rates of frontotemporal dementia, primary progressive aphasia, and semantic dementia in the U.S. and world population are unknown. However, one study reviewed medical records from 1,683 patients at a large Veteran's Affairs Medical Center Memory Disorders clinic over a 4-year period. The study was the largest to date on early onset dementia and the authors reported an unexpectedly large number of patients who were below the age of 65 and had with cognitive deficits (30% of all patients). Frontotemporal dementia was the leading cause of dementia not attributable to preventable causes, such as alcohol abuse. This contrasted with the causes of late-onset dementia where Alzheimer's disease prevailed (McMurtray et al., 2006). A similar study from Japan also concluded that early-onset dementia is not rare and that the clinical characteristics and causes of early onset dementia differed from late onset dementia. In a sample of 668 demented patients, 28% were early onset cases, with frontotemporal dementia as a leading cause of dementia in this group (Shinagawa et al., 2007). While the exact rates of the other dementia syndromes, besides Alzheimer's disease, in the general population are not known, it is becoming increasingly clear that approximately 1/3 of dementia cases present before the age of 65 and in most cases the predominant cause of the dementia in all age groups is something other than Alzheimer's disease, and often have aphasia as a key symptom.

Degenerative Dementias with Presenile Onset and Aphasia

Arnold Pick was the first to report of a patient with progressive aphasia (loss of the ability to produce and/or comprehend language) and this report was the basis of the concept of Pick's disease (Pick, 1892). In his report, he described the aphasia as being caused by a single circumscribed atrophic process in the brain and established the concept of focal atrophy causing a specific behavioral syndrome. Today, Pick's disease is often reserved for the pathological description of frontotemporal atrophy with silver staining, globular inclusions (Pick bodies), swollen neurons (Pick cells), superficial cortical spongiosis, neuronal loss and gliosis (Kertesz, 2001). However, these diagnostic criteria present some difficulties. First, the pathologic findings are only known at autopsy, which is clearly not helpful to the clinician faced with a symptomatic patient. Second, only 25% of cases have the typical inclusions. To address these challenges, patients with focal atrophy are better described by their clinical presentation, such as the specific aspects of aphasia. Furthermore, it is now understood that although some cases have Pick bodies, the majority do not, and the clinical syndrome is not affected by the pathological variant. There are several clinical presentations that are widely described. A patient with a primarily apathy - disinhibition dementia is said to have Frontotemporal Dementia (FTD) or Frontotemporal Dementia – frontal variant (FTD-fv), since the focal atrophy is largely in the frontal lobes. A patient with a progressive aphasia is said to have Primary Progressive Aphasia (PPA) or Frontotemporal Dementia – temporal variant, since the focal atrophy is in the temporal lobes. A patient with loss of meaning and words is said to have Semantic Dementia (SD) and the atrophy is often initially in the left temporal lobe. There is considerable overlap in all three conditions and over time, patients acquire the symptomatology of another condition as atrophy spreads. Thus, a patient that starts with FTD may eventually develop the aphasia of PPA or a patient that initially presents with PPA may develop the disinhibition characteristic of FTD (Blair et al., 2007; Kertesz, 2001; Marczinski et al., 2004).

Age of onset for FTD, PPA, and SD is most commonly between 45 and 65 years (Neary & Snowden, 1996). In general, a family history of a similar disorder in a first-degree relative occurs in approximately half of cases (Neary & Snowden, 1996) and familial cases tend to have an earlier onset (Kertesz & Munoz, 2002). There are case reports of very young onset in patients who were age 25 (Coleman et al., 2002) and 27 (Jacob et al., 1999) when diagnosed with FTD. Unfortunately, optimal treatment for FTD, PPA and SD has been difficult to establish and just like with AD, there is no known cure. Failures to recognize the widespread existence of these conditions have potentially contributed to the slow emergence of effective treatments.

Diagnosis of these early onset dementias is challenging. Often, the characteristic clinical findings often lead individuals to be inappropriately treated as depressed before considering referral to a neurologist. However, there are some indications that specific cognitive tasks, such as category and letter fluency tasks, and specific behavioral assessments, such as the Frontal Behavioral Inventory, may be more helpful in distinguishing various early onset dementia syndromes from normal controls and from one another (Diehl et al., 2005; Marczinski et al., 2004; Marczinski & Kertesz, 2006). The rest of this chapter will describe these lesser-known dementia syndromes in greater detail, and will then present new ways to distinguish these various syndromes from one another.

Frontotemporal Dementia (FTD)

The core symptoms of Frontotemporal Dementia (FTD) are personality change, apathy, blunting of emotions, lack of insight, and disinhibition (Brun et al., 1994). Other symptoms include loss of personal hygiene, loss of social awareness, hypersexuality, hyperorality, perseverative behavior, utilization behavior (i.e., excessive touching), and distractibility. Affective symptoms include indifference, remoteness, inertia and aspontaneity (Kertesz et al.,

1997). Early diagnosis of FTD can be extremely difficult because cognitive functioning may be initially well preserved in these patients. Any poor performance on psychometric tests is often due to the patient being uncooperative or easily distracted when given task instructions. Psychiatric symptoms may predate the onset of FTD by many years (Neary & Snowden, 1996). The hallmark feature of disinhibition can range from childish rude behavior to kleptomania. Patients can come in contact with the law when they steal, grope strangers or expose themselves. The social inappropriateness frequently makes family members uncomfortable and embarrassed. Hypersexuality may only be verbal or gestural in the middle-aged patient. Hyperorality often manifests as overeating or development of food fads, particularly for things like sweets. As atrophy is occurring in the frontal lobes, some executive dysfunction is evident in psychometric testing. However, for the most part, cooperative patients, despite their grossly abnormal behavior, can perform well on most psychometric tests (Kertesz & Munoz, 2002). If the disease has progressed, aphasia may be present (Blair et al., 2007).

Primary Progressive Aphasia (PPA)

Primary Progressive Aphasia (PPA) is characterized by an isolated and gradual dissolution of language function. PPA symptoms start with anomia (word finding difficulty), progress to a loss of fluency, and are ultimately followed by mutism (Kertesz et al., 2003; Mesulam, 1987). Anomia is also a feature of Alzheimer's Disease. Therefore, the operational definition of PPA includes a period of two years of progressive aphasia with relative preservation of other functions and activities of daily living (Weintraub et al., 1990). Even in fully mute patients, relatively well-preserved memory and visuospatial orientation is often evident and PPA patients may function surprisingly well in the community if they do not start developing the disinhibition of FTD when atrophy spreads from the temporal lobes into the frontal lobes (Kertesz & Munoz, 2002).

Semantic Dementia (SD)

Semantic Dementia (SD) is characterized by a pattern of profound deterioration of semantic memory that disrupts the meaning, recognition, and comprehension of objects (Hodges et al., 1992; Snowden et al., 1989). For example, a patient may no longer know what a 'steak', a 'tool' or a 'vehicle' is (Kertesz et al., 1998). This lexicosemantic language impairment is in striking contrast to the relatively preserved phonological and syntactic process of language and cognition in general (Hodges et al., 1994). In other words, patients can speak fluently and coherently, yet they have lost the meaning of some words. The lexical and semantic aspects of the representation progressively deteriorate in a frequency dependent manner, with the loss of lower frequency words first (e.g., the word 'antelope' is lost before the word 'dog'). However, with disease progression, higher frequency words become increasingly lost (Bird et al., 2000). The neuropsychological profile of patients with SD contrasts greatly with other dementias (such as AD), as the patients have well-preserved episodic memory and visuospatial skills (Graham & Hodges, 1997).

Alzheimer's Disease (AD)

In contrast to FTD, PPA and SD described above, the core features of AD include episodic memory deficits and visual-spatial deficits (Hodges et al., 1999; Storey et al., 2002). While episodic memory deficits are often severe in AD, more subtle impairments in semantic memory and visuospatial skills are often observed (Hodges et al., 1999). The other dementias are difficult to distinguish from AD clinically because AD exists in several variants. A patient can present with a predominant impairment of executive, visuospatial, or language skills (Storey et al., 2002). Word finding difficulties in AD are often present, at times quite early on in the disease process (Appell et al., 1982). However, aphasia in AD is associated with a more advanced disease process. Symptoms might include impairments in articulation, repetition of words, fluency, animal naming, and confrontational naming (Coen et al., 1996; Weiner et al., 20008). Impaired verbal and semantic fluency have been documented in AD patients compared to age-matched controls (Chertkow & Bub, 1990; Diaz et al., 2004; Duff Canning et al., 2004; Forbes-McKay et al., 2005; Henry et al., 2004; Martin & Fedio, 1983; Nebes, 1989). Structural imaging in AD generally shows global cortical atrophy, including hippocampal atrophy (Black, 1996), compared to the focal frontal and temporal atrophy seen in patients with FTD, PPA and SD (Kertesz et al., 1997).

General Cognitive Testing

In the assessment of various degenerative dementias, the examination of cognition is often carried out with brief psychometric tests. The Mini-Mental Status Examination (MMSE) has been shown to be a useful and highly popular instrument (Folstein, Folstein & McHugh, 1975). Since this short test includes questions that query orientation (what is the date today?) and visuospatial skills (draw a clock), results from the MMSE often identify quickly when AD is a possibility. However, this test is often insensitive to the earliest changes in individuals with dementia, particularly in high-functioning and/or highly educated individuals. Especially early in the disease process, patients may compensate for their aphasia by selecting other words, slowing down their speech, or using other strategies. Furthermore, the MMSE and even longer mental status exams, such as the Mattis Dementia Rating Scale (MDRS) (Mattis, 1988), have been shown to fail to distinguish between various degenerative dementias, such as AD, FTD, PPA and SD (Kertesz et al., 2003). As such, clinicians have sought better diagnostic neuropsychological assessments that still incorporate brevity as a key feature necessary for administration in a clinical setting.

Diagnostic Utility of Fluency Measures

Verbal fluency tasks consist of generating words from a semantic category (e.g., animals) or words beginning with a given letter (e.g. letter 'S') with a specified time limit, such as 60 seconds. While both categories and letter fluency task performance is impaired by degenerative dementias, there are some differences in performance between these two tasks, suggesting that letter and category fluency tasks rely on both some common and some distinct cognitive processes (Pompeia et al., 2002; Rende et al., 2002). It has been suggested that the category tasks may rely more heavily on access to lexical representations of semantic concepts, whereas the letter task may rely more heavily on the central executive component of working memory (Baddeley, 1992; Baddeley et al., 1975), and this distinction appears to have anatomical correlates (Gold & Buckner, 2002).

Category and letter fluency tasks have been used for several decades to determine if dementia is present in a patient. For example, AD patients perform worse on both types of fluency tasks compared to normal controls suggesting that these brief tests can identify when a disease process is present. Furthermore, word fluency performance may be an early predictor of rate of progression in AD, as poor performance indicates that the disease is more advanced (Coen et al., 1996). However, more recently, it has been suggested that these brief tests may also be helpful in distinguishing various dementia syndromes from one another, and not just from controls. Duff Canning et al. (2004) published the first study to suggest the utility of category and letter fluency tasks in distinguishing dementia syndromes from one another. The authors compared patients with AD to patients with vascular dementia (VaD) and normal controls. The one-minute category task involved naming as many animals as possible. The one-minute letter fluency task involved naming as many words that began with the letter 'F' as possible. The authors reported that both patient groups generated fewer animal names compared to normal elderly controls. Furthermore, letter fluency scores differentiated AD from VaD, with patients with AD able to generate more 'F' words compared to patients with VaD.

The success of this approach led to the suggestion that the fluency test might be a powerful test to aid in diagnostic decisions, and could be deemed the one-minute mental status examination (Cummings, 2004). The appeal of the fluency task as a one-minute mental status exam is that it is extremely brief to administer while yielding tremendously rich data. For instance, patients' responses can provide several pieces of information such as: (1) the raw number of words generated with the one minute trial, (2) the actual word frequencies of the words generated, based on published norms of the English language, and (3) the numbers of errors made of repeating a word within the one minute trial. Duff Canning et al. (2004) only reported the raw number of words produced by the patients in the trial. However, it has been hypothesized that this potential rich data may be useful in distinguishing the various degenerative dementias with aphasia that pose diagnostic dilemmas for clinicians (Marczinski & Kertesz, 2006). For instance, the number of errors of repetition (where there is at least one intervening item) could indicate deficits of working memory. Imagine two patients who both score 7 on the animal task. The first patient has a response list of 'giraffe, cow, dog, cat, lion, beaver, snake' while the second patient has a response list of 'dog, cow, horse, dog, sheep, snake, dog'. Clearly, the two lists are not equal. The second patient demonstrates a deficit in working memory in that the patient 'forgets' that he has already produced a particular exemplar from a category. By only scoring raw numbers of words produced, this important memory error is not captured. Furthermore, word frequencies indicate access to lexical representations with impairment indicated by failures to generate lower frequency exemplars. For example, a generated three word animal list of zebra, squirrel, and frog, includes lower frequency exemplars from the English language in comparison to a generated three word animal list of horse, dog, and bear. Again, while matched in the number of words generated, the two lists are qualitatively difference in access to lexical representations.

With this new approach, performance on category and letter fluency tasks was compared in patients with SD, PPA and AD (Marczinski & Kertesz, 2006). While it could easily be predicted that all these dementia patients would perform more poorly on both types of fluency tasks compared to normal elderly controls, more specific predictions about differences in performance between the groups could be made. Since profound deterioration of semantic memory is the key feature in SD, SD patients would be expected to produce the fewest number of words in a category task and produce more words in a letter task that relies more on the central executive component of working memory. Furthermore, the words generated in the category task should be higher in word frequency, since the lower word frequency words have been lost due to the disease process. Finally, errors of repeating a word within a list would be expected to occur very infrequently in patients with SD, as they characteristically have well-preserved working memory and would be less likely than AD patients to forget that they had just generated a particular exemplar from a category within a one minute trial.

Since verbal fluency is significantly impaired in PPA, it could be predicted that patients with PPA would produce the fewest number of words in both the category and letter fluency tasks. In particular, letter fluency might be dramatically impaired as patients with PPA have a deficit in accessing phonemes (the sound-based representation of speech) (Mendez et al., 2003). The mean word frequencies produced should be lower in PPA compared to SD patients, as the disease process of PPA impairs speech production more than access to lexical representations (e.g., a patient with PPA is more likely to produce a low frequency exemplar like antelope than a patient with SD). Furthermore, errors or repeating words within a list would be unlikely, as episodic and working memory remains relatively intact in patients with PPA.

As the core features of AD include episodic memory deficits and visual-spatial deficits, performance on fluency tasks should contrast greatly to the performance of patients with PPA and SD. Impaired verbal and semantic fluency has been documented in AD patients compared to controls (Chertkow & Bub, 1990; Diaz et al., 2004; Duff Canning et al., 2004; Martin & Fedio, 1983; Nebes, 1989). Low letter fluency scores discriminate AD patients from controls and are a reliable predictor of subsequent dementia status in elderly patients (Hodges & Patterson, 1994). However, results from previous studies would suggest that AD patients would generate more words in category and letter tasks compared to PPA patients (Kertesz et al., 2003; Mendez et al., 2003). Mean word frequencies should be lower in AD compared to SD, as semantic retrieval deficits are primary in SD and secondary in AD (Hodges et al., 1999). Finally, errors of repeating words within a list should be most impaired in AD as the disease process results in impairments in episodic memory.

Research Strategy

The aim of the following study was therefore to demonstrate that the category and letter fluency tasks distinguish patients with SD, PPA, and AD from controls and from one another (see Marczinski & Kertesz, 2006). Three fluency tasks (two category fluency tasks of animals and groceries and one letter fluency task of words that start with the letter S) were administered. For animal category fluency, participants were asked to name as many different animals as they could within 60 seconds. For grocery category fluency, participants were instructed to name as many different items that they might purchase in the grocery store as they could within 60 seconds. Instructions emphasized that they should name individual items and not just a category label such as meat. For 'S' words letter fluency, participants were asked to name as many different words that start with the letter 'S' as they could within 60 seconds. Instructions emphasized that words generated should not include proper names such as Sally. Responses were tape-recorded and each word was generated was then assigned its appropriate word frequency based on the Kucera-Francis word frequency norms (Kucera & Francis, 1967). An error was recorded if the individual repeated a word within a list. From these verbatim responses, there were three dependent measures of interest: (1) the number of words generated, (2) the mean word frequency of the words generated, and (3) the number of errors of repetition divided by the total number of words generated. Thus, the current methodology used in fluency tasks was expanded upon for this study. By recording word frequencies, one might have more information about the status of lexical representations of semantic concepts. By recording the number of errors made, one might have more information about the status of episodic memory.

Study Participants

Twenty clinically diagnosed AD patients, 8 clinically diagnosed SD patients, 12 clinically diagnosed PPA patients, and 20 normal elderly controls participated in this study. The demographic characteristics of these groups are presented in Table 1. The clinical diagnosis was made according to the criteria suggested for AD by the National Institute of Neurological Communicative Disorders and Stroke-Alzheimer's disease and Related Disorders Association (NINCDS-ADRDA) (McKhann et al., 1984), SD by Neary et al. (1988), and PPA by Mesulam (1987). Diagnostic decisions were made independent of fluency scores. Spouses and caregivers were recruited as normal control participants if they were healthy individuals older than 65 years of age without any history of psychiatric or neurological disease.

Results

Fluency task performance differed as predicted (see Marczinski & Kertesz, 2006). As shown in Figure 1, controls generated the most exemplars in all three fluency tasks, followed by AD, SD and PPA patients. Interestingly, SD and PPA patients did not differ statistically for the two category fluency tasks. By contrast, AD and SD did not differ from one another on the letter fluency task.

Table 1. Means (M) and standard deviations (SD) of various demographic characteristics of patients and controls.

	Controls		Alzheimer's disease (AD)		Semantic Dementia (SD)		Primary Progressive Aphasia (PPA)		
	M	*SD*	*M*	*SD*	*M*	*SD*	*M*	*SD*	*Sign.*
Sample size (N)	20		20		8		12		
Gender (M:F)	10:10		10:10		4:4		6:6		.99
Age at test (yrs)	73.8	5.9	74.7	7.6	65.9	9.3	63.1	7.1	<.001
Age of onset (yrs)	n/a		71.5	7.0	61.9	9.7	59.4	7.5	<.001
Duration ill (yrs)	n/a		3.2	2.3	4.0	2.1	3.5	1.6	.63
Education (yrs)	13.5	2.8	9.9	3.0	14.0	3.4	14.1	2.7	<.001
MMSE	28.8	1.1	21.3	4.0	22.6	8.6	15.3	6.5	<.001
MDRS	137.7	4.3	111.9	11.7	102.4	27.9	74.6	32.8	<.001

Note: MMSE = Mini Mental Status Exam; MDRS = Mattis Dementia Rating Scale.

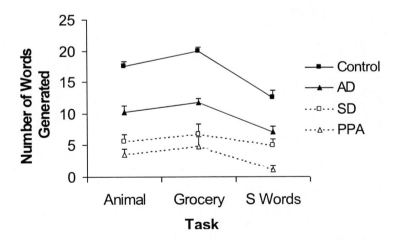

Figure 1. Mean number of words generated in the animal, grocery and 'S' words fluency tasks for controls, patients with Alzheimer's disease, patients with Semantic Dementia, and patients with Primary Progressive Aphasia. Error bars reflect standard errors of the mean.

Significant differences in the patient groups were obtained for the mean word frequency of the words generated in the animal and grocery category tasks. Figure 2 illustrates that the controls generated the lowest frequency exemplars in the animal task, followed by AD, PPA and SD patients. For the grocery task, a slightly different pattern emerged as AD patients generated words with higher mean word frequencies compared to all other groups. There were no significant differences between the groups for the mean word frequency from the S letter task.

The proportion of repetition errors generated in the animal category task revealed a significant difference between groups. Figure 3 illustrates that AD patients generated more errors compared to the other three groups. PPA and SD patients made no repetition errors on any of the three tasks. There were no significant differences found in the proportion of errors generated in the grocery category or the S letter task.

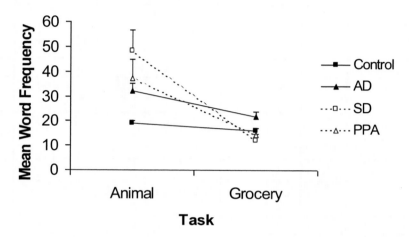

Figure 2. Mean word frequencies of words generated in the animal and grocery fluency tasks for controls, patients with Alzheimer's disease, patients with Semantic Dementia, and patients with Primary Progressive Aphasia. Error bars reflect standard errors of the mean.

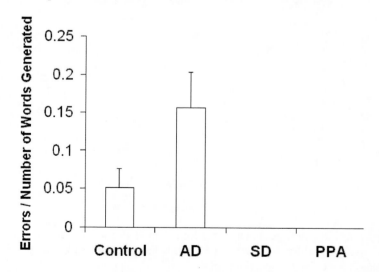

Figure 3. Mean number of perseveration errors divided by the total number of words generated in the animal fluency task for controls, patients with Alzheimer's disease, patients with Semantic Dementia, and patients with Primary Progressive Aphasia. None of the patients with Semantic Dementia or Primary Progressive Aphasia made any errors in this task. Error bars reflect standard errors of the mean.

Summary of the Study Results

The results provide support for the hypothesis that category and letter fluency tasks can be used to distinguish various dementia syndromes from normal controls and from one another. All patient groups generated fewer words in all three tasks (animals, groceries, 'S' words) compared to normal controls. In all three tasks, AD patients generated the most exemplars, followed by the SD and PPA patients, consistent with hypotheses regarding the extent of language involvement in these three conditions. The category tasks did not differentiate the SD and PPA patients. However, the SD patients generated more exemplars in the letter task compared to the PPA patients, which further supports the phonological impairment in PPA in contrast to the semantic deficit in SD. When the mean word frequencies of the words generated were compared for the animal task, controls generated lower frequency exemplars, followed by AD, PPA and then SD patients generating the higher frequency exemplars, as predicted. Surprisingly, this pattern was not replicated in the grocery task where the higher frequency exemplars were generated by the AD patients. Finally, errors of repeating a word within a list in the animal category task were significantly higher for the AD patients compared to all other groups, as hypothesized based on deficits in short term working memory.

Importance of the Findings

Accurate diagnosis for degenerative diseases with aphasia is critical for identifying diseases early and making appropriate treatment decisions. Recently, verbal fluency has been shown to be impaired in mild cognitive impairment (MCI) compared to age-matched controls (Murphy et al., 2006; Nutter-Upham et al., 2008). Since MCI is a high-risk factor for AD, these simple fluency tasks may be an easy way to identify preclinical dementia populations (Murphy et al., 2006). Some researchers have suggested that verb fluency is an even better linguistic marker for incipient dementia, compared with letter or noun fluency (Ostberg et al., 2005).

There are a number of diverse interventions that are available to treat aphasia (Hillis, 2007). While effective pharmacotherapy for aphasia for these various syndromes is still a work in progress, some potentially useful drug therapies have been reported (de Boissezon et al., 2007). For example, patients with PPA show language improvements on the drug galantamine (Freedman, 2007). In a recent clinical trial, patients with PPA who were treated with galantamine had language scores that remained stable throughout the drug trial, whereas patients with PPA who were treated with a placebo showed deterioration that was typical of the disease process (Kertesz et al., 2008). In addition, any pharmacotherapy for aphasia in dementia appears more effective when the drug treatment coincides with speech therapy (de Boissezon et al., 2007). Other novel treatments are also on the horizon. Spinal administration of etanercept, a TNF-alpha inhibitor that acts by blocking the binding of this cytokine to its receptors, has shown efficacy for both AD and PPA. A recent study determined whether perispinal etanercept had the potential to improve verbal function in AD. They observed that this treatment improved language skills in AD patients over the six month clinical trial

(Tobinick et al., 2008). Besides pharmacotherapy, other novel approaches are on the horizon. Transcranial magnetic stimulation (TMS) may be useful for aphasic patients (Devlin & Watkins, 2007).

Conclusion

Distinguishing between the various degenerative dementias where aphasia can be present in varying degrees has long posed significant diagnostic challenges to the clinician. As the population ages and the numbers of patients with new onset of dementia symptoms rise, clinicians will increasingly require efficient and effective methods for distinguishing between these dementia syndromes to provide accurate and timely diagnosis and treatment. Through a better understanding of the clinical and pathological distinctions between these syndromes, it has been possible to develop and test a novel method for using previously established category and letter fluency tasks to generate new data that can be used to help clinicians faced with this problem. Through not only recording the number of words generated, but also recording word frequencies and repetition errors, patients with Alzheimer's Disease can now be differentiated from those with Semantic Dementia and Primary Progressive Aphasia. The ability to make such distinctions despite modest sample sizes and the use of only three fluency tasks provides great encouragement for the possible future benefit of this new methodology. Within the time constraints of a screening assessment in a neurological clinic, the category and letter fluency tasks may therefore provide the clinician key information to allow quick and accurate diagnosis, and ultimately better access to appropriate treatment for this difficult group of diseases.

References

Andreasen, N., Blennow, K., Sjodin, C., Winblad, B. & Svardsudd, K. (1999). Prevalence and incidence of clinically diagnosed memory impairments in a geographically defined general population in Sweden. The Pitea Dementia Project. *Neuroepidemiology, 18*, 144-155.

Appell, J., Kertesz, A. & Fisman, M. (1982). A study of language functioning in Alzheimer patients. *Brain and Language, 17*, 73-91.

Ayyagari, P., Salm, M. & Sloan, F. A. (2007). Effects of diagnosed dementia on Medicare and Medicaid program costs. *Inquiry, 44*, 481-494.

Baddeley, A. (1992). Working memory. *Science, 255*, 556-559.

Baddeley, A. D., Thomson, N. & Buchanan, M. (1975). Word length and the structure of short-term memory. *Journal of Verbal Learning and Verbal Behaviour, 14*, 575-589.

Bird, H., Lambon Ralph, M. A., Patterson, K. & Hodges, J. R. (2000). The rise and fall of frequency and imageability: Noun and verb production in semantic dementia. *Brain and Language, 73*, 17-49.

Black, S. E. (1996). Focal cortical atrophy syndromes. *Brain and Cognition, 31*, 188-229.

Blair, M., Kertesz, A., McMonagle, P., Davidson, W. & Bodi, N. (2006). Quantitative and qualitative analyses of clock drawing in frontotemporal dementia and Alzheimer's disease. *Journal of the International Neuropsychological Society, 12*, 159-165.

Blair, M., Marczinski, C. A., Davis-Faroque, N. & Kertesz, A. (2007). A longitudinal study of language decline in Alzheimer's disease and frontotemporal dementia. *Journal of the International Neuropsychological Society, 13*, 237-245.

Brun, A., Englund, B., Gustafson, L., et al. (1994). Clinical and neuropathological criteria for frontotemporal dementia. *Journal of Neurology Neurosurgery and Psychiatry, 57*, 416-418.

Chertkow, H. & Bub, D. (1990). Semantic memory loss in dementia of Alzheimer's type. What do various measures measure? *Brain, 113*, 397-417.

Coen, R. F., Maguire, C., Swanwick, G. R., Kirby, M., Burke, T., Lawlor, B. A., Walsh, J. B. & Coakley, D. (1996). Letter and category fluency in Alzheimer's disease: a prognostic indicator of progression? *Dementia, 7*, 246-250.

Coleman, L. W., Digre, K. B., Stephenson, G. M. & Townsend, J. J. (2002). Autopsy-proven, sporadic pick disease with onset at age 25 years. *Archives of Neurology, 59*, 856-859.

Cummings, J. L. (2004). The one-minute mental status examination. *Neurology, 62*, 534-535.

de Boissezon, X., Peran, P., de Boysson, C. & Demonet, J. F. (2007). Pharmacotherapy for aphasia: myth or reality? *Brain and Language, 102*, 114-125.

Devlin, J. T. & Watkins, K. E. (2007). Stimulating language: insights from TMS. *Brain, 130*, 610-622.

Diaz, M., Sailor, K., Cheung, D. & Kuslansky, G. (2004). Category size effects in semantic and letter fluency in Alzheimer's patients. *Brain and Language, 89*, 108-114.

Diehl, J., Monsch, A. U., Aebi, C., Wagenpfeil, S., Krapp, S., Grimmer, T., Seeley, W., Forstl, H. & Kurz, A. (2005). Frontotemporal dementia, semantic dementia, and Alzheimer's disease: the contribution of standard neuropsychological tests to differential diagnosis. *Journal of Geriatric Psychiatry and Neurology, 18*, 39-44.

Duff Canning, S. J., Leach, L., Stuss, D., Ngo, L. & Black, S. E. (2004). Diagnostic utility of abbreviated fluency measures in Alzheimer disease and vascular dementia. *Neurology, 62*, 556-562.

Feldman, H. & Kertesz, A. (2001). Diagnosis, classification and natural history of degenerative dementias. *Canadian Journal of Neurological Sciences, 28 Supplement 1*, S17-S27.

Folstein, M. F., Folstein, S. E. & McHugh, P. R. (1975). 'Mini-Mental State': A practical method for grading the cognitive state of patients for the clinician. *Journal of Psychiatric Research, 12*, 189-198.

Forbes-McKay, K. E., Ellis, A. W., Shanks, M. F. & Venneri, A. (2005). The age of acquisition of words produced in a semantic fluency task can reliably differentiate normal from pathological age related cognitive decline. *Neuropsychologia, 43*, 1625-1632.

Freedman, M. (2007). Frontotemporal dementia: recommendations for therapeutic studies, designs, and approaches. *Canadian Journal of Neurological Sciences, 34 Suppl 1*, S118-S124.

Graham, K. S. & Hodges, J. R. (1997). Differentiating the roles of the hippocampal complex and the neocortex in long-term memory storage: Evidence from the study of semantic dementia and Alzheimer's disease. *Neuropsychology, 11*, 77-89.

Gustafson, L. (1987). Frontal lobe degeneration of non-Alzheimer type, II: clinical picture and differential diagnosis. *Archives of Gerontology and Geriatrics, 6*, 209-223.

Gustafson, L. (1993). Clinical picture of frontal lobe degenerescence of non-Alzheimer type. *Dementia, 4*, 143-148.

Hebert, L. E., Scherr, P. A., Bienias, J. L., Bennett, D. A. & Evans, D. A. (2003). Alzheimer disease in the US population. *Archives of Neurology, 60*, 1119-1122.

Heidler-Gary, J., Gottesman, R., Newhart, M., Chang, S., Ken, L. & Hillis, A. E. (2007). Utility of behavioral versus cognitive measures in differentiating between subtypes of frontotemporal lobar degeneration and Alzheimer's disease. *Dementia Geriatric and Cognitive Disorders, 23*, 184-193.

Henry, J. D., Crawford, J. R. & Phillips, L. H. (2004). Verbal fluency performance in dementia of the Alzheimer's type: a meta-analysis. *Neuropsychologia, 42*, 1212-1222.

Heston, L. L. & Mastri, A. R. (1982). Age at onset of Pick's disease and Alzheimer's dementia: implications for diagnosis and research. *Journal of Gerontology, 37*, 422-424.

Hillis, A. E. (2007). Aphasia: progress in the last quarter of a century. *Neurology, 10*, 200-213.

Hodges, J. R. & Patterson, K. (1994). Is semantic memory consistently impaired early in the course of Alzheimer's disease? Neuroanatomical and diagnostic implications. *Neuropsychologia, 4*, 441-459.

Hodges, J. R., Patterson, K. & Tyler, L. K. (1994). Loss of semantic memory: Implications for the modularity of mind. *Cognitive Neuropsychology, 11*, 505-542.

Hodges, J. R., Patterson, K., Oxbury, S. & Funnell, E. (1992). Semantic dementia. Progressive fluent aphasia with temporal lobe atrophy. *Brain, 115*, 1783-1806.

Hodges, J. R., Patterson, K., Ward, R., Garrard, P., Bak, T., Perry, R. & Gregory, C. (1999). The differentiation of semantic dementia and frontal lobe dementia (temporal and frontal variants of frontotemporal dementia) from early Alzheimer's disease: a comparative neuropsychological study. *Neuropsychology, 13*, 31-40.

Jacob, J., Revesz, T., Thom, M. & Rossor, M. N. (1999). A case of sporadic Pick disease with onset at 27 years. *Archives of Neurology, 56*, 1289-1291.

Jobst, K. A., Barnetson, L. P. & Shepstone, B. J. (1997). Accurate prediction of histologically confirmed Alzheimer's disease and the differential diagnosis of dementia: the use of NINCDS-ADRDA and DSM-III-R criteria, SPECT, X-ray CT, and APO E4 medial temporal lobe dementias. The Oxford Project to Investigate Memory and Aging. *International Psychogeriatrics, 9 Supplement 1*, 191-222.

Kertesz, A. (1979). *Aphasia and Associated Disorders: Taxonomy, Localization, and Recovery.* New York, NY: Grune & Stratton.

Kertesz, A. (2001). Pick's disease. *The Canadian Journal of Continuing Medical Education, September*, 141-155.

Kertesz, A. (2006). *Western Aphasia Battery – Revised.* Pearson.

Kertesz, A. & Munoz, D. G. (2002). Frontotemporal dementia. *Medical Clinics of North America, 86*, 501-518.

Kertesz, A. & Poole, E. (2004). The aphasia quotient: the taxonomic approach to measurement of aphasic disability. 1974. *Canadian Journal of Neurological Sciences, 31*, 175-184.

Kertesz, A., Davidson, W. & Fox, H. (1997). Frontal behavioral inventory: Diagnostic criteria for frontal lobe dementia. *Canadian Journal of Neurological Sciences, 24*, 29-36.

Kertesz, A., Davidson, W. & McCabe, P. (1998). Primary progressive semantic aphasia: A case study. *Journal of the International Neuropsychological Society, 4*, 388-398.

Kertesz, A., Davidson, W., McCabe, P., Takagi, K. & Munoz, D. (2003). Primary progressive aphasia: Diagnosis, varieties, evolution. *Journal of the International Neuropsychological Society, 9*, 710-719.

Kertesz, A., Morlog, D., Light, M., Blair, M., Davidson, W., Jesso, S. & Brashear, R. (2008). Galantamine in frontotemporal dementia and primary progressive aphasia. *Dementia and Geriatric Cognitive Disorders, 25*, 178-185.

Knopman, D. S. (2001). An overview of common non-Alzheimer dementias. *Clinical Geriatric Medicine, 17*, 281-301.

Kucera, H. & Francis, W. N. (1967). *Computational Analysis of Present-day American English.* Providence, RI: Brown University Press.

Marczinski, C. A. & Kertesz, A. (2006). Category and letter fluency in semantic dementia, primary progressive aphasia, and Alzheimer's disease. *Brain and Language, 97*, 258-265.

Marczinski, C. A., Davidson, W. & Kertesz, A. (2004). A longitudinal study of behavior in frontotemporal dementia and primary progressive aphasia. *Cognitive and Behavioral Neurology, 17*, 185-190.

Martin, A. & Fedio, P. (1983). Word production and comprehension in Alzheimer's disease: The breakdown of semantic knowledge. *Brain and Language, 19*, 124-141.

Mattis, S. (1988). *Dementia rating scale.* Odessa, FL: Psychological Assessment Resources Professional manual.

McMurtray, A., Clark, D. G., Christine, D. & Mendez, M. F. (2006). Early-onset dementia: frequency and causes compared to late-onset dementia. *Dementia Geriatric and Cognitive Disorders, 21*, 59-64.

Mendez, M. F., Clark, D. G., Shapira, J. S. & Cummings, J. L. (2003). Speech and language in progressive nonfluent aphasia compared with early Alzheimer's disease. *Neurology, 61*, 1108-1113.

Mesulam, M. M. (1987). Primary progressive aphasia – differentiation from Alzheimer's disease. *Annals of Neurology, 22*, 533-534.

Murphy, K. J., Rich, J. B. & Troyer, A. K. (2006). Verbal fluency patterns in amnestic mild cognitive impairment are characteristic of Alzheimer's type dementia. *Journal of the International Neuropsychological Society, 12*, 570-574.

Neary, D. & Snowden, J. (1996). Fronto-temporal dementia: Nosology, neuropsychology, and neuropathology. *Brain and Cognition, 31*, 176-187.

Neary, D., Snowden, J. S. & Mann, D. M. A. (1993). The clinical pathological correlates of lobar atrophy. *Dementia, 4*, 154-159.

Neary, D., Snowden, J. S., Bowen, J. S., et al. (1986). Neuropsychological syndromes in presenile dementia due to cerebral atrophy. *Journal of Neurology Neurosurgery and Psychiatry, 49*, 163-174.

Nebes, R. D. (1989). Semantic memory in Alzheimer's disease. *Psychology Bulletin, 106*, 377-394.

Nutter-Upham, K. E., Saykin, A. J., Rabin, L. A., Roth, R. M., Wishart, H. A., Pare, N. & Flashman, L. A. (2008). Verbal fluency performance in amnestic MCI and older adults with cognitive complaints. *Archives of Clinical Neuropsychology, 23*, 229-241.

Ostberg, P., Fernaeus, S. E., Hellstrom, K., Bogdanovic, N. & Wahlund, L. O. (2005). Impaired verb fluency: a sign of mild cognitive impairment. *Brain and Language, 95*, 273-279.

Ostbye, T., Taylor, D. H., Clipp, E. C., Van Scoyoc, L. & Plassman, B. L. (2008). Identification of dementia: Agreement among national survey data, Medicare claims, and death certificates. *Health Services Research, 43*, 313-326.

Pasquier, F. (1999). Early diagnosis of dementia: neuropsychology. *Journal of Neurology, 246*, 6-15.

Perry, R. J. & Hodges, J. R. (2000). Differentiating frontal and temporal variant frontotemporal dementia from Alzheimer's disease. *Neurology, 54*, 2277-2284.

Pick, A. (1892). Uber die beziehungen der senilen hirnatrophie zur aphasie. *Prag Med Wochenschr, 17*, 165-167.

Pompeia, S., Rusted, J. M. & Curran, H. V. (2002). Verbal fluency facilitated by the cholinergic blocker, scopolamine. *Human psychopharmacology, 17*, 51-59.

Rende, B., Ramsberger, G. & Miyake, A. (2002). Commonalities and differences in the working memory components underlying letter and category fluency tasks: A dual-task investigation. *Neuropsychology, 16*, 309-321.

Roth, H. L. & Heilman, K. M. (2000). Aphasia: A Historical Perspective. In S.E. Nadeau, B.A. Crosson, & L. Gonzalez-Rothi (Eds.), *Aphasia and Language: Theory to Practice*. New York, NY: Guildford Press.

Shewan, C. M. & Kertesz, A. (1980). Reliability and validity characteristics of the Western Aphasia Battery (WAB). *Journal of Speech and Hearing Disorders, 45*, 308-324.

Shinagawa, S., Ikeda, M., Toyota, Y., Matsumoto, T., Matsumoto, N., Mori, T., Ishikawa, T., Fukuhara, R., Komori, K., Hokoishi, K. & Tanabe, H. (2007). Frequency and clinical characteristics of early-onset dementia in consecutive patients in a memory clinic. *Dementia Geriatric and Cognitive Disorders, 24*, 42-47.

Snowden, J. S. & Neary, D. (1993). Progressive language dysfunction and lobar atrophy. *Dementia, 4*, 226-231.

Snowden, J. S., Goulding, P. J. & Neary, D. (1989). Semantic dementia: A form of circumscribed cerebral atrophy. *Behavioral Neurology, 2*, 167-182.

Storey, E., Slavin, M. J. & Kinsella, G. J. (2002). Patterns of cognitive impairment in Alzheimer's disease: assessment and differential diagnosis. *Frontiers in Bioscience, 7*, e155-e184.

Tobinick, E. L. & Gross, H. (2008). Rapid improvement in verbal fluency and aphasia following perispinal etanercept in Alzheimer's disease. *BMC Neurology, 21*, 27.

Weiner, M. F., Neubecker, K. E., Bret, M. E. & Hynan, L. S. (2008). Language in Alzheimer's disease. *Journal of Clinical Psychiatry, 69*, 1223-1227.

Weintraub, S., Rubin, N. P. & Mesulam, M. M. (1990). Primary progressive aphasia: Longitudinal course, neuropsychological profile, and language features. *Archives of Neurology, 47*, 1329-1335.

Wichlund, A. H., Johnson, N. & Weintraub, S. (2004). Preservation of reasoning in primary progressive aphasia: further differentiation from Alzheimer's disease and the behavioral presentation of frontotemporal dementia. *Journal of Clinical and Experimental Neuropsychology, 26*, 347-355.

In: Aphasia: Symptoms, Diagnosis and Treatment
Editors: G. Ibanescu, S. Pescariu

ISBN: 978-1-60741-288-5
© 2009 Nova Science Publishers, Inc.

Chapter IV

Real-Time Comprehension in Agrammatic Aphasia

Petra B. Schumacher

Max Planck Institute for Psycholinguistics, Nijmegen, the Netherlands and
Johannes Gutenberg University Mainz, Germany

Abstract

In recent years, the availability of online techniques (i.e., when language comprehension is measured as a sentence unfolds) has given rise to a new line of research complementing traditional findings from offline methodologies and providing finer-grained characterizations of the deficit underlying aphasia. The emerging data question the classic characterization of the agrammatic aphasia comprehension deficit as one of loss of certain structural representations. The present chapter thus provides a review of a slowly but steadily growing body of experimental research into the real-time sentence processing of individuals with agrammatic Broca's aphasia. It draws on evidence that mainly derives from the comprehension of various non-canonical structures (including *wh*-questions, passives, cleft constructions, and NP-movement) as well as pronominal interpretation, and that is based on data from cross-modal lexical decision priming and interference tasks, anomaly detection, word monitoring paradigms, eye tracking and electrophysiology. The chapter discusses the implications of these real-time data for theoretical accounts of the aphasic syndrome and argues for slowed-down processing rather than loss of knowledge representations as the sources of the comprehension deficit.

Introduction

Brain injury caused by cerebrovascular insults, trauma or infections often results in an inability to produce and/or comprehend language properly. Different forms of this loss of language ability (aphasia) emerge depending on the area and size of the brain injury. One particular type of aphasia, known as agrammatism, is characterized by telegraphic speech on the side of language production (i.e., effortful speech and short utterances that lack functional categories, such as articles or tense markers) and a specific deficit targeting syntactic relations on the side of language comprehension. This loss of specific language capacities often coincides with brain injury in Broca's area (Brodmann Areas 44 and 45) and the regions surrounding it in the left inferior frontal cortex as well as the underlying white matter.

In this chapter, I will focus on the *comprehension deficit* in agrammatism. People with agrammatism have difficulties comprehending sentences that deviate from the unmarked structure (such as subject-before-object order in English) or more generally that depend on certain dependency relations between phrase structural information units for full interpretation. This has led researchers to characterize the agrammatic deficit as syntactic in nature. To illustrate this, consider the following examples:

1.   The boy pushed the girl.
2.   The girl was pushed by the boy.

While people with agrammatism correctly interpret the sentence in (1) as the boy performing a pushing-action on the girl, they are unable to determine who is the pusher (the agent of the action) and who is being pushed (the undergoer of the action) in the example sentence provided in (2). When, for instance, presented with a picture selection task consisting of a picture that shows a girl pushing a boy and another picture that shows a boy pushing a girl, agrammatic patients perform at chance level and select both the structurally correct and incorrect picture about 50% of the time. This comprehension deficit is attributed to an inability to properly establish syntactic dependency relations because the structure in (2) can be derived from that in (1) via a syntactic operation that promotes the undergoer of an action (the one who was pushed) to the sentence-initial subject position (which serves as unmarked position for the agent of an action). The distinction between the sentences in (1) and (2) is also discussed with respect to canonicity, since the former structure represents the canonical word order and the latter passive sentence the non-canonical word order. Crucial for present purposes is that non-canonical sentences are more demanding in terms of sentence processing because they enhance structural complexity, and that these structures are especially vulnerable in the agrammatic system.

Early aphasia research has viewed agrammatism as a loss of syntactic information [cf. Grodzinsky, 2000 for a comprehensive overview of offline data from a variety of different languages and sentential environments]. Within this line of thinking, some researchers have argued that the syntactic trace—a phonologically unrealized copy of a displaced constituent—cannot be accessed any longer in the agrammatic system [Grodzinsky, 2000] or that the indices that connect a dislocated element with its trace are no longer represented [Mauner, Fromkin, & Cornell, 1993], while others have claimed that the construction of the syntactic representation is impaired to the extent that certain syntactic projections cannot be represented any longer [Friedmann & Grodzinsky, 1997]. However, the growing body of evidence from online sentence comprehension suggests that the knowledge that is required to interpret an utterance like (2) is not lost, but that certain operations are impeded and delayed due to limited processing resources [e.g., Swinney & Zurif, 1995; Piñango, 2000; Avrutin, 2006]. Such a delay allows other potential interpretations to emerge, for instance, on the basis of heuristic strategies like "the first noun phrase in a sentence represents the agent, i.e., the one who carries out an action", which then compete with the untimely occurring syntax-based interpretation (i.e., the first noun phrase represents the undergoer of the action).

In the following section, I provide a brief overview of evidence for a resource-based deficiency in agrammatism and sketch a model of sentence comprehension that considers slowed-down processing as the cause of the agrammatic comprehension deficit. In subsequent sections, I review online data from sentence comprehension in agrammatism that represent a variety of linguistic phenomena, including pronoun interpretation, *wh*-movement, argument movement, and anomaly detection, and it will be demonstrated how aphasia research has benefited from the development and application of online methodologies. At the same time, it will be shown how the different findings can be accounted for in terms of a slowed-down processing account, and how this, together with the emergence of alternative compensatory interpretations, can explain the divergence between online and offline findings that sometimes seem to indicate a decline in language proficiency across time (from good online performance to chance-level offline performance in, for instance, object relative sentences). Corroborating support for a particular functional specification of the left inferior frontal cortex on the basis of neuroimaging data will also be briefly touched upon, as well as the fact that agrammatic comprehension mirrors processes that can emerge in the intact processing system as well, albeit under specific circumstances (e.g., time pressure or special registers) and as suboptimal processing routes. The present chapter does not discuss potential effects of general working memory capacity and task demands [cf., e.g., Love, Haist, Nicol, & Swinney, 2006; Caplan, Waters, Dede, Michaud, & Reddy, 2007]. Although these factors might impact sentence comprehension in the agrammatic system, the data discussed in this chapter indicate that they are not exclusively contributing to the deficit and that a more specific characterization of the agrammatic syndrome can be put forth.

Agrammatism as a Resource Limitation

Finding out more about the time-course of processing is highly relevant for accounts that view the agrammatic deficit as a limitation of processing capacity. Such a resource limitation may coincide with slow activation rates of different types of linguistic information [as suggested by Haarmann & Kolk, 1991 and Friederici & Kilborn, 1989] and/or fast decay rates of specific linguistic knowledge [see Haarmann & Kolk, 1994], but it could also be connected to a more general limitation of working memory capacity [e.g., Caplan et al., 2007]. Utilizing a cross-modal syntactic priming paradigm, Friederici and Kilborn [1989] varied the inter-stimulus interval between the offset of an auditorily presented sentence fragment and the onset of a visually presented target word. Participants were instructed to make a lexical decision to the visually presented target string (i.e., does the string represent a word or a non-word in the language under investigation?). When given a longer inter-stimulus interval of 200 ms (vs. no inter-stimulus interval), agrammatic patients showed faster response times, lending initial support to the claim that temporal constraints induce the agrammatic comprehension deficit and cause slow activation. Haarmann and Kolk [1994] applied a word monitoring task, in which participants first saw a target word and then heard a sentence that did or did not contain an agreement violation; the participants' task was to press a button as soon as they detected the target word. There was an effect of the agreement mismatch with no inter-stimulus interval, but this effect diminished with an inter-stimulus interval of 750 ms—while it was retained in the neurologically intact control group— indicating that the relevant linguistic information had already decayed in the agrammatic system. Haarmann and Kolk further suggested that agrammatic comprehension is restricted by both slow activation and fast decay, but that only one of these limitations takes place at a time.

The goal of more recent research has been to narrow down the actual cause of this processing deficit. Past research indicated that the comprehension difficulties of agrammatic patients can be closely tied to an inability to properly implement specific linguistic information. On the basis of real-time comprehension data, it has been proposed that the *processing resources needed to implement syntactic knowledge* are limited in the agrammatic system, resulting in a slowing down of syntactic structure building. If this is the correct account of the agrammatic deficit, then all operations depending on the timely formation of syntactic structure should be impaired (at least temporarily). At the same time that syntactic structure formation is delayed, competing sources of (extra-syntactic) information become available [cf. Piñango, 2000, 2002; Avrutin, 2004, 2006]. Yet, once syntactic representations are built, the coexistence of two competing interpretations—one guided by late syntactic information, the other by extra-syntactic considerations—results in guessing, as evidenced by distinct performance patterns in offline tasks [see for instance Piñango, 2002; Avrutin, 2006; Ruigendijk, Vasic, & Avrutin, 2006; and the discussion of compensatory interpretations below]. How such a slowing down of syntactic structure formation affects different sentence types and processing decisions is detailed in the following sections.

Syntactic Movement

Many syntactic theories rely on movement operations to derive sentence structures from their unmarked (i.e., canonical) counterparts [e.g., Chomsky, 1981]. A moved constituent leaves behind a placeholder at the base position that remains phonologically unrealized (referred to as trace or t in the following). This is illustrated in (3) (indeces ($_i$) are used in the examples to mark the dependency between a moved constituent and its trace). The trace in turn is the entity that receives thematic role assignment from the verb (e.g., agent or undergoer of an action), and therefore a link between the trace and the displaced constituent is required to transfer the thematic role information to the moved constituent.

3.   The girl$_i$ was pushed t$_i$ by the boy.

Lexical priming studies have shown that the meaning of a displaced constituent is reactivated at the position of the trace and crucially not at an earlier point, indicating that activation of a lexical meaning decays over time, but can be reactivated at the trace position [e.g., Nicol & Swinney, 1989]. Priming refers to the observation that lexical decisions are faster to a word that is related to a previously processed word than to a word that is semantically unrelated to previously processed information. The underlying logic is that the previously processed word (e.g., *girl*) is (re)activated by a semantically related word (e.g., *dress*), but unaffected by an unrelated word (e.g., *desk*), and that this activation lowers the recognition threshold of the target word (yielding faster reaction times).

Interestingly, in contrast to neurologically unimpaired participants, agrammatic patients do not show reactivation patterns at the trace position [Zurif, Swinney, Prather, Solomon, & Bushell, 1993; Swinney, Zurif, Prather, & Love, 1996], but priming effects occur further downstream at a later point in time [cf. Love, Swinney, & Zurif, 2001; Burkhardt, Piñango, & Wong, 2003; Love, Swinney, Walenski, & Zurif, 2008]. These latter studies employed the cross-modal lexical decision priming paradigm, where participants perform two tasks: listening to a sentence for comprehension and making a lexical decision to a visually presented letter string (i.e., does the letter string represent a real word of the language under investigation or a non-word?). Response times to related (e.g., for (4) *fighter*) and unrelated words (e.g., *climber*) presented at different positions throughout the sentence (indicated by ①, ②, etc., below) are then compared.

4. The audience liked the wrestler$_i$ ① that the ② parish priest condemned t$_i$ ③ for ④ foul ⑤ language.

In sentences like (4), unimpaired comprehenders show priming effects (i.e., faster response times to related words) immediately after the critical word (①) and at the trace position (③). In contrast, agrammatic comprehenders show delayed priming effects (at ② and ⑤, respectively) [Love et al., 2001, 2008]. These findings suggest that the structural representations of the dependencies between displaced constituents and their traces become available in the agrammatic system at some point during online processing, and this is taken as evidence for slower-than-normal sentence comprehension in agrammatism.[6] The cross-modal priming data from Burkhardt et al. [2003] substantiate the processing delay hypothesis on the basis of relative clause constructions similar to (4) and structures as in (5) which are also considered to undergo syntactic movement. The latter represent an instance of so-called unaccusative constructions, in which the argument of the verb (*butter*) is base-generated in post-verbal position (*t*), but is moved to the sentence-initial position for the language-specific requirement to have a pre-verbal noun phrase. In these unaccusative structures, unimpaired

---

[6] Blumstein, Byma, Kurowski, Hourihan, Brown, & Hutchinson [1998] seem to provide counter-evidence for this processing delay claim. Using a uni-modal lexical decision priming paradigm, their participants heard both auditorily presented sentences (that contained a displaced constituent) and auditorily presented targets for the lexical decision task, and they reported close to normal priming effects for the agrammatic participant group. However, the decisive difference to the priming studies outlined above was that the critical trace positions were at (or very close to) the end of a sentence (e.g., *The president visited the city$_i$ that the big earthquake destroyed t$_i$.*), and as a consequence Blumstein et al. might have measured end-of-sentence wrap-up effects (which are subserved by semantic- and discourse-level processing) rather than evidence for the establishment of a dependency between a displaced constituent and its trace. See Balogh, Zurif, Prather, Swinney, & Finkel [1998] for support for separable demands on dependency formation and end-of-sentence wrap-up and a detailed discussion of why Blumstein et al.'s data should not be taken to oppose the findings from slowed down sentence processing.

participants showed priming effects only at position ③, while a later priming effect (at ④) was again registered for agrammatic participants.[7]

5.   The butter$_i$ in the small white dish ① melted t$_i$ ② after the ③ boy ④ turned on the microwave.

These priming data suggest that agrammatic patients are able to form dependencies between moved constituents and their base positions (traces) but in a temporally protracted manner. The patients appear to lack sufficient processing resources to form dependencies within the typical time course parameters, which results in later than normal priming patterns (specifically, a temporal delay of about 150–550 ms was observed compared to the unimpaired system). However, an intriguing discrepancy remains between the delayed online patterns and offline data. While typical priming effects occur with a temporal delay (suggesting that the underlying representations have been properly formed), the offline performance of agrammatic patients still shows deficient sentence comprehension, reflected in chance performance on picture matching tasks or acting-out tasks. This discrepancy can be accounted for by a clash of conflicting interpretations: In the absence of timely structure build-up, alternative strategies are recruited to reach an interpretation (e.g., heuristics as described above that assign an agent role to the first noun phrase or the use of information from a different linguistic domain, such as discourse representation). By the time the delayed syntax-based interpretation becomes available, it competes with the alternative interpretation, yielding chance performance in offline tasks [cf., e.g., Piñango, 2000; Avrutin, 2006; and further discussions below].

Previous findings from a visual world paradigm seem to weaken these claims about slower-than-normal processing [Dickey, Choy, & Thompson, 2007]. Agrammatic patients were asked to listen to brief stories that ended in an object-*wh*-question (e.g., *Who did the boy kiss that day at school?*) while they looked at a visual display with three related images (*boy, girl, school*) and a distractor image (*door*):

6.   This story is about a boy and a girl. One day, they were at school. The girl was pretty, so the boy kissed the girl.
Who$_i$ did the boy kiss t$_i$ that day at school?

Eye fixations on the different images were calculated and revealed that agrammatic participants looked at the object image (*girl*) at the position of the trace approximately as often as neurologically unimpaired participants. This was taken as evidence for the timely establishment of a syntactic dependency between the displaced constituent and its trace. However, it should be noted that comprehension difficulties do generally not arise with *who-*

---

[7] The fact that relative clause traces (as in (4)) show priming immediately at the trace position, while noun phrase traces (5) show later priming effects in the unimpaired system is due to differences in the underlying syntactic structures. Relative clause traces (wh-traces) have been reported to have more immediate reactivation patterns than noun phrase traces (NP-traces) [cf. Nicol and Swinney, 1989], possibly because the relative pronoun creates an expectation for a trace (i.e., the parser actively searches for a trace position), and this cue is absent

questions as attested by offline comprehension tasks [Hickok & Avrutin, 1996] and that the visual display might have encouraged looks to the target for independent reasons. Moreover, as observed by Love et al. [2008], the sentences were presented at a slower-than-normal rate (3.3 syllables per second), and such a slowing down of the speech input has recently also resulted in improved comprehension patterns in agrammatic patients [cf. Love et al., 2008]. See below for further details about the influence of the rate of presentation on sentence comprehension in both the agrammatic and the unimpaired processing system.

Non-Movement-Based Dependencies: Pronoun Resolution

Agrammatic patients also show atypical comprehension patterns during pronoun resolution, a phenomenon that is not based on syntactic movement and is not subject to the canonicity distinction, but still requires the formation of a dependency (between the pronominal and its antecedent). In (7), the reflexive *himself* can only refer to *the skier*, but not to *the boxer*, while the pronoun *him* in (8) refers to *the boxer*, but not to *the skier*. These different readings for reflexives and pronouns are governed by principles that depend on proper structural representations and that require a local antecedent for reflexives and a non-local antecedent for pronouns.

7. The $boxer_i$ said that the $skier_k$ in the hospital had blamed $himself_k$ ① for the recent injury.
8. The $boxer_i$ said that the $skier_k$ in the hospital had blamed him_i ① for the recent injury.

In offline tasks, agrammatic individuals comprehended reflexives in a relatively normal fashion, while pronoun interpretation was rather defective [cf., e.g., Grodzinsky, Wexler, Chien, Marakovitz, & Solomon, 1993; Piñango, 2002; Ruigendijk et al., 2006]. In contrast, online tasks reveal that agrammatic comprehenders encounter difficulties during the real-time implementation of reflexive-antecedent dependencies, but resolve them further downstream, while the comprehension problems with pronoun-antecedent dependencies remain. More specifically, while unimpaired participants show priming for the structurally correct antecedent right at the pronominal element (e.g., *snow* yields priming effects at the reflexive in (7), but not at the pronoun in (8)), a cross-modal lexical decision priming study with agrammatic participants reported no priming for reflexives immediately after the reflexive [Love, Nicol, Swinney, Hickok, & Zurif, 1998]. Love and colleagues auditorily presented sentences as in (7) above and the participants were asked to listen to these sentences and perform a lexical decision task to a visually presented word. Lexical decision times to a related word (such as *snow*) were not significantly faster than those to an unrelated word when measured right after the reflexive (① above). This indicated that the reflexive-

---

in the case of NP-movement. Crucially, however, agrammatic patients show overall delays in both time course patterns.

antecedent dependency had not been formed yet. In sentences such as (8), the patients showed aberrant priming (faster responses to a word like *snow* that primes the structurally unavailable antecedent *the skier*), suggesting that both reflexive-antecedent and pronoun-antecedent relations are affected by lesions to the left inferior frontal cortex. Overall, the study revealed an intriguing discrepancy between online and offline data, where across time, comprehension of reflexives improves, while pronoun interpretation is poor across the board. Yet, the study did not probe priming at a later point in time, which could provide immediate support for a slower-than-normal processing account.

However, evidence from investigations using the cross-modal lexical decision interference task shed light on pronominal comprehension further downstream. In this task, sentences are also presented auditorily and a lexical decision task to a visually presented target has to be carried out. However, in contrast to the priming paradigm, the lexical decision is made to a semantically unrelated word. Response times to this lexical decision reflect processing cost arising from the listening comprehension task. The underlying logic is that the same processing resources are recruited for the two tasks, and that enhanced computational demands in the listening task should result in higher response times in the lexical decision task. In addition, this task measures processing cost exerted by distinct linguistic domains, e.g., when interpretation depends on information from distinct linguistic domains, enhanced processing demands (i.e., higher response times) are predicted to emerge. This paradigm was employed to probe the interpretation patterns of two types of pronominals that have the same form but are subject to processes in two distinct linguistic domains: while the interpretation of the reflexive in (9) is considered to be based on syntactic information, the reflexive in (10) requires additional extra-syntactic information for interpretation. Note that the reflexive in (10) is often referred to as 'logophor' and represents a pronominal form that refers to an individual whose perspective, point of view or thoughts are conveyed. Accordingly, it has been claimed that logophors depend on extra-syntactic (discourse) information to fully account for these additional interpretive properties of point of view. For more detailed theoretical characterizations, see, for instance, Hagège, 1974; Zribi-Hertz, 1989; Sells, 1987; or Burkhardt, 2005 for an extensive overview.

9. The detective$_i$ who was famed ① disguised himself$_k$ ② before the ③ undercover investigation started at dawn.

10. The climber$_i$ buckled a belt ① around himself$_k$ ② before the ③ group set out for the strenuous ascent.

Neurologically intact participants show interference (i.e., significantly higher response times) immediately after the reflexive in (10) compared to (9), indicated by ② in the examples above, and at none of the other positions [Burkhardt, 2005]. Research with agrammatic patients revealed no interference effects at this position (②). Instead higher response times were measured further downstream at position ③, indicating again that normal processing patterns occur with a temporal delay in the agrammatic system [see Burkhardt, 2005 and Burkhardt, Avrutin, Piñango, & Ruigendijk, 2008 for evidence from English and Dutch]. Moreover, this delay was attributed to slowed-down syntactic processing, since syntactic information must be fully available before the domain where interpretation takes place can be determined (i.e., the question of whether there is a potential local antecedent for the reflexive or not). This appears to be the case further downstream, about 500 ms later than in the intact processing system, where 'normal' interference effects emerged.

Anomaly Detection

A discrepancy also emerges between comprehension patterns and grammaticality judgments. In spite of their interpretation problems, people with agrammatism perform rather well on grammaticality judgment tasks. When asked to judge the grammaticality of certain sentence structures in offline tasks, agrammatic patients show a high degree of sensitivity with respect to the acceptability and unacceptability of sentence structures. The research literature reports on a variety of syntactic violations—including movement-based violations (e.g., violations relating to subject-auxiliary inversion, particle movement, relative clause movement) as well as non-movement-based violations (e.g., violations of phrase structure or subcategorization principles, agreement errors)—that were detected with a high degree of accuracy by the agrammatic participants [see, for instance, Linebarger, Schwartz, & Saffran, 1983; Shankweiler, Crain, Gorrell, & Tuller, 1989; Wulfeck, Bates, & Capasso, 1991]. Sample violations are given in the a)-cases of (11) to (16) from Linebarger et al. [1983] and Wulfeck et al. [1991]. Nevertheless, these patients presented with the typical comprehension problems in offline picture matching or acting-out tasks, and this dissociation may be attributed to task-specific demands, since potential alternative interpretations may not weigh that heavily during grammaticality judgments. Alternatively, grammaticality decisions and comprehension processes may be subserved by distinct neural subsystems (see below for neuroimaging evidence).

11. a *He came my house at six o'clock. (subcategorization violation)
   b He came to my house at six o'clock.
12. a *The gift my mother is very nice. (phrase structure violation)
   b The gift for my mother is very nice.
13. a *He are picking the last apple from the large tree. (agreement violation)
   b He is picking the last apple from the large tree.
14. a *Is the boy is having a good time? (subject-auxiliary
   b Is$_i$ the boy t$_i$ having a good time?   inversion violation)
15. a *How many did you see birds in the park? (left branching violation)
   b How many birds$_i$ did you see t$_i$ in the park?
16. a *Mary ate the bread that I baked a cake? (filled relative clause gap
   b Mary ate the bread$_i$ that I baked t$_i$?   violation)

Online measures substantiate the agrammatic patients' high sensitivity in judgment tasks. In early investigations of sentence processing under temporal restrictions, participants listened to sentences and had to indicate whether a sentence was good or bad by pressing a response button as soon as possible, which (should have) yielded grammaticality judgments before the end of the sentence. Agrammatic participants again showed above chance sensitivity to the critical manipulations, albeit with overall slower response times compared to an unimpaired control group—which, however, could have been caused by more general (motor skill) deficits [Wulfeck et al., 1991; Lu, Bates, Li, Tzeng, Hung, Tsai, Lee, & Chung, 2000].

However, all of these anomaly and ungrammaticality detection tasks provide rather coarse-grained measures (compared to eye-tracking data or electrophysiological measures, but also to cross-modal priming and interference tasks) and response times in these stop-making-sense tasks are even registered after the end of the sentence. Therefore alternative measures are more auspicious for real-time investigations of sentence comprehension in agrammatism. Electrophysiological recordings provide one means of assessing more fine-grained temporal parameters of sentence comprehension and have been used extensively to investigate linguistic violations. Research with neurologically unimpaired participants has for instance revealed that subcategorization violations (similar to the example violation in (11.a) above) evoke an early negative-going electrophysiological deflection that has its maximum over left anterior electrode sites. In a single-case study with an agrammatic patient who had to listen to sentences and make a sentence-final grammaticality judgment, no such effect for early phrase structure building was registered (while other electrophysiological responses were spared), supporting the view that basic syntactic structure formation is vulnerable in the agrammatic system [Friederici, Hahne, & von Cramon, 1998]. Note that grammaticality judgments were nevertheless at ceiling level, converging with the observations outlined above. Further investigations with neurologically intact participants have shown that agreement mismatches (similar to (13.a) above) are generally reflected by a positive-going electrophysiological deflection peaking around 600 ms after the onset of the mismatching word (so-called P600 component). Contrary to this, agrammatic patients as a group are reported to lack such an electrophysiological response to agreement violations [Hagoort, Wassenaar, & Brown, 2003]. Note, however, that this absence of the effect was driven by agrammatic patients who presented with a severe impairment (based on offline measures of individual syntactic performance) and that the electrophysiological responses were modulated by the severity of the impairment: participants with a severe deficit did not show electrophysiological correlates of the agreement violation, while mildly impaired participants elicited a reduced positivity compared to the unimpaired controls. This reduction in the amplitude of the electrophysiological signal might be taken as evidence for reduced processing resources.

Evidence from Neuroimaging

The data from online comprehension in agrammatism discussed thus far indicate that damage to the left inferior frontal cortex disrupts certain syntax-dependent operations. Neuroimaging research with neurologically unimpaired participants supports this functional characterization and provides more precise localization value for the cortical areas engaged in sentence processing.

Using functional magnetic resonance imaging, numerous studies have shown that differences in syntactic complexity are reflected in modulations of the hemodynamic responses in left inferior frontal brain regions (Broca's area) [Just, Carpenter, Keller, Eddy, & Thulborn, 1996; Röder, Stock, Neville, Bien, & Rösler, 2002; Ben-Shachar, Palti, & Grodzinsky, 2004; Friederici, Fiebach, Schlesewsky, Bornkessel, & von Cramon, 2006; among many others]. In contrast, the processing of syntactically ungrammatical sentences (in comparison to their grammatical counterparts) has been shown to activate brain regions in the left posterior frontal operculum (among others) [e.g., Friederici, Rüschemeyer, Hahne, & Fiebach, 2003; Friederici et al., 2006]. For instance, Friederici and colleagues [2006] report that syntactic complexity (defined over varying numbers of movement operations within a sentence) was modulated by activation in a subarea of Brodmann Area 44 (the inferior portion of the left pars opercularis); crucially, ungrammatical utterances showed activation in the left deep posterior frontal operculum (which is adjacent to Brodmann Area 44), indicating that processes associated with complexity and ungrammaticality are subserved by distinct brain regions [for an overview of corroborating findings see Friederici, 2004]. This dissociation might also explain the different behavioral patterns in grammaticality judgments and comprehension questions respectively, and it gives rise to the prediction that the left posterior frontal operculum should be spared in those agrammatic patients who present with good performance in grammaticality judgment tasks.

On Compensation and Alternative Routes of Interpretation

Thus far, the data from aphasia research as well as neuroimaging studies suggest that left inferior frontal brain regions are involved in interpretative processes that are contingent on syntactic structure formation. In particular, the online data indicate that access to or use of this information is protracted, and crucially not lost (contra to what some theories have proposed in the past). However, agrammatic patients show both improvement and decay of comprehension across time, and this puzzling observation demands an explanation. For instance, while reflexive elements do not show immediate reactivation patterns at the reflexive itself, evidence for the establishment of reflexive-antecedent dependencies surfaces with a 500 ms temporal delay; and this improvement remains in responses to offline truth-value judgment tasks. Similarly, displaced constituents in object relative clauses do not show reactivation patterns at the trace position, but further downstream, again around 500 ms later than in the intact system; however, this progress is not evident in offline tasks where chance performance is observable. This selective dissociation triggering good online performance and poor offline performance in some cases has been explained in terms of competing routes of interpretation.

First of all, agrammatic patients appear to compensate for their (initial) comprehension deficit by recruiting information from other linguistic domains [e.g., Caramazza & Zurif, 1976; Kolk, 2000; Avrutin, 2006; Piñango, 2006]. For instance, Avrutin [2006] suggests that people with agrammatism recruit extra-syntactic information (such as contextual or information structural knowledge) because syntax is too weak to provide sufficient information for interpretation. Another compensatory strategy relies on world knowledge and general expectations that can guide sentence interpretation beyond syntactic reasoning, as exemplified by different response patterns to semantically reversible and irreversible sentences [e.g., Caramazza & Zurif, 1976]. As outlined above, agrammatic comprehenders may also rely on a heuristic strategy that is based on the linear ordering of arguments and assigns an actor role to the first argument of a sentence [cf., e.g., Grodzinsky, Piñango, Zurif, & Drai, 1999; Piñango, 2006]. Second, these alternative interpretations become available while syntactic information is not available yet because the processing system strives for a fast and automatic interpretation at any given point in time. However, once syntactic representations are built further downstream, a conflict arises between the two sources of interpretation (if they differ from each other). To illustrate this, consider the case of object relative clauses as in (17). The linear order heuristics (i.e., agent before undergoer) would assign the thematic role of agent to the first-mentioned noun phrase (*the girl*) and the role of undergoer to *the boy*. Syntactic information in turn would identify *the boy* as the agent and *the girl* as the undergoer (via thematic role assignment by the verb). When these two interpretations clash further downstream, the comprehender does not know which one to choose and chance performance arises. Such a clash does not occur in the intact system, because syntactic representations are considered most economical and powerful.

17. The girl$_I$ who the boy pushed t$_i$ was blond.

The fact that reflexive interpretation is initially vulnerable but ultimately surfaces with good comprehension has been explained by a bias induced by the truth-value judgment tasks used in the offline experimentations. The picture or the objects/puppets used in the acting-out task provide another cue for interpretation, which facilitates the correct reading in some cases resulting in above-chance performance [see Piñango, 2002 for a detailed discussion of competing interpretations during pronoun resolution]. Electrophysiological data also seem to suggest that agrammatic comprehenders revert to extra-syntactic information in the absence of sufficient syntactic support, as evidenced by the emergence of a semantics-related electrophysiological signature (enhanced N400 component) in response to phrase-structure violations (where neurologically intact participants elicited a syntax-related P600 signature) [Hagoort et al., 2003].

To conclude this discussion of competing information, in many languages, syntactic information takes precedence over alternative interpretations that are based on the compensation strategies outlined above and this is so for reasons of economy. However in the agrammatic system, syntactic information is not readily available to be powerful enough to override these alternative routes. As a consequence, false interpretations can arise during agrammatic comprehension. Interestingly, some of these strategies and alternative routes are also employed in the unimpaired system. Under certain circumstances, the normal comprehender may have to, and is able to, interpret a sentence that lacks certain syntactic information—consider for instance newspaper headlines or, formerly, telegrams that typically lack tense or case information [cf., e.g., Tesak & Dittmann, 1991]. This phenomenon implies that agrammatic comprehenders revert to processes that are also available in the intact system, which however do not represent the most economical routes and therefore only occur under very restricted conditions in the neurologically intact system.

On Timely Availability

The evidence presented thus far supports the view that the agrammatic comprehension deficit results from a processing limitation that prevents the timely allocation of certain linguistic knowledge. Another important finding with respect to the time course of sentence comprehension is the observation that slowing down the presentation rate of the input yields improved comprehension patterns in agrammatic patients [e.g., Love et al., 2008]. Love and colleagues carried out a series of experiments utilizing the cross-modal lexical decision priming paradigm as well as the (offline) sentence-picture matching paradigm and varied the presentation rate of auditorily presented sentences (normal rate of 4.5 syllables per second vs. slow rate of 3.4 syllables per second). Agrammatic patients showed reliably improved comprehension in the slowed down presentation mode, evidenced by correct priming as early as at the trace position in object relative sentences and enhanced accuracy rates in the picture verification task. The latter finding indicates that alternative interpretations lose their impact on the comprehension decisions when the speech input is presented at a slower than normal rate thus making available the relevant (and most economical) interpretive route. In contrast, time manipulations in investigations with neurologically unimpaired participants (here, slowing down the presentation rate of the input), aggravated performance. Similarly, exerting time pressure on unimpaired control participants yielded deficient comprehension [David Swinney, personal communication]. These data generally substantiate the claim that temporal factors impact sentence comprehension, which in turn indicates that the observed patterns are closely tied to processing resources. It further demonstrates that the patterns in agrammatic comprehenders mirror certain processes that can take place in the intact system as well.

Conclusion

In light of the observations presented in this chapter, the comprehension deficit in agrammatism should be characterized as a processing limitation targeting syntactic structure building: agrammatic comprehension fails whenever the underlying syntactic representation is unable to properly constrain the possible interpretations that the processing system can contemplate for a given sentence. Evidence for a limitation of processing resources advancing syntactic structure formation (and contra loss of linguistic knowledge) comes from real-time investigations of sentence comprehension that reveal slower than normal processing patterns across various experimental paradigms. The online evidence generally indicates that the temporal parameters of agrammatic comprehension differ from comprehension in the intact system in such a way that the typical experimental effects—like reaction times in priming or interference tasks or eye movements—are observable with a temporal delay (ranging between 150–550 ms after the critical point in unimpaired processing). And this delay emerges for sentences whose interpretation depends exclusively on syntactic information, such as long-distance dependencies in object relative sentences and passives, pronominal relations or phrase structure relations.

It is not entirely clear yet whether the capacity limitation affects operations on syntactic representations proper or the speed of lexical retrieval, which is a prerequisite for complete structure building. A weaker explanation of the slow down hypothesis views lexical operations as the source of slowed down processing in agrammatism [cf., e.g., Prather, Zurif, Love, & Brownell, 1997]. Under this view, syntactic structure formation is slowed down because it depends on the timely availability of lexical information. On the word level, Prather and colleagues [1997] showed with a list priming task that slowing down the presentation rate improved lexical decision accuracy in agrammatic patients, who showed priming with 1500 ms inter-stimulus intervals—while unimpaired age-matched participants already showed priming effects with an inter-stimulus interval of 500 ms. On the sentence level, Love et al. [2008] demonstrated that slowing down the speech rate (to 3.4 syllables per second compared to a typical rate of 4.5 syllables per second) yielded priming effects at the critical trace position for agrammatic participants. More generally, the research on lexical-semantic processing in agrammatism indicates that agrammatic patients show typical lexical priming effects in word lists and sentential contexts with overall longer response latencies [e.g., Prather et al., 1997; Kiran & Thompson, 2003; Myers & Blumstein, 2005]. Yet, in contrast to lexical-semantic relations, selectional restrictions (e.g., the kind of arguments a verb takes) appear to be more susceptible to comprehension deficits, possibly because they are qualitatively different or because they are not couched within a rich network of associations [cf. Myers & Blumstein, 2005]. Accordingly, slowed down activation or, more specifically, access to selectional features might impact syntax-dependent comprehension.

However, such a lexical-based explanation of the slow down in agrammatism cannot account for the fact that slowing differentially affects certain sentence structures. In general, we observe a certain degree of gradience, i.e., some constructions are comprehended better than others. For instance, local dependencies show a processing advantage over more distant dependencies [as, for instance, exemplified by word monitoring data from subcategorization violations vs. long-distance dependencies in Baum, 1989 or the priming data from noun phrase- and *wh*-movement of Burkhardt et al., 2003]. In this latter case, distinct delay latencies were reported for *wh*-movement and noun phrase movement (550 ms vs. 150 ms, respectively—using the same participants), which can be explicated if distinct syntactic operations are assumed for these two types of dependencies. In addition, it has been claimed that these effects are not driven by pure distance (i.e., attributable to a short-term memory deficit) but can be ascribed to the underlying syntactic manipulations. A processing advantage for 'simpler' structures has also been observed in real-time investigations with neurologically intact comprehenders [e.g., Friederici et al., 2006].

Overall, aphasia research can benefit from the growing body of research on real-time comprehension patterns since it adds a critical dimension—time course data—to the characterization of the deficit and has therefore important implications for the development of therapeutic tools. While offline results represent the combination of a multiplicity of processes interacting with each other during sentence comprehension, online measures have the advantage of tapping into fast and automatic processes at various points during the construction of meaning, hence providing a finer-grained window into successful as well as deficient language processing. Given the rising sophistication in online experimentation, these methodologies are also capable of identifying the specific linguistic domains implicated by a certain deficit. Together with the localization data from neuroimaging studies, a more consistent understanding of sentence comprehension in agrammatism—as well as in the neurologically intact system—can thus be obtained.

References

Avrutin, S. (2004). Optionality in Child and Aphasic Speech. *Lingue e Linguaggio*, *3(1)*, 65-95.

Avrutin, S. (2006). Weak syntax. In: Y. Grodzinsky, & K. Amunts (Eds.), *Broca's region* (49-62). Oxford: Oxford University Press.

Balogh, J., Zurif, E., Prather, P., Swinney, D. & Finkel, L. (1998). Gap-filling and end-of-sentence effects in real-time language processing: Implications for modeling sentence comprehension in aphasia. *Brain and Language*, *61(2)*, 169-182.

Baum, S. R. (1989). Online sensitivity to local and long-distance syntactic dependencies in Broca's aphasia. *Brain and Language*, *37(2)*, 327-338.

Ben-Shachar, M., Palti, D. & Grodzinsky, Y. (2004). Neural correlates of syntactic movement: converging evidence from two fMRI experiments. *Neuroimage*, *21(4)*, 1320-1336.

Blumstein, S. E., Byma, G., Kurowski, K., Hourihan, J., Brown, T. & Hutchinson, A. (1998). On-line processing of filler-gap constructions in aphasia. *Brain and Language*, *61(2)*, 149-168.

Burkhardt, P. (2005). *The syntax-discourse interface: Representing and interpreting dependency*. Amsterdam/Philadelphia: John Benjamins.

Burkhardt, P., Avrutin, S., Piñango, M. M. & Ruigendijk, E. (2008). Slower-than-normal syntactic processing in agrammatic Broca's aphasia: Evidence from Dutch. *Journal of Neurolinguistics*, *21(2)*, 120-137.

Burkhardt, P., Piñango, M. M. & Wong, K. (2003). The role of the anterior left hemisphere in real-time sentence comprehension: Evidence from split intransitivity. *Brain and Language*, *86(1)*, 9-22.

Caplan, D., Waters, G., Dede, G., Michaud, J. & Reddy, A. (2007). A study of syntactic processing in aphasia I: Behavioral (psycholinguistic) aspects. *Brain and Language*, *101(2)*, 103-150.

Caramazza, A. & Zurif, E. B. (1976). Dissociation of algorithmic and heuristic processes in language comprehension: Evidence from aphasia. *Brain and Language*, *3(4)*, 572-582.

Chomsky, N. (1981). *Lectures on government and binding*. Dordrecht; Cinnaminson: Foris.

Dickey, M. W., Choy, J. W. J. & Thompson, C. K. (2007). Real-time comprehension of wh-movement in aphasia: Evidence from eyetracking while listening. *Brain and Language*, *100(1)*, 1-22.

Friederici, A. D. & Kilborn, K. (1989). Temporal constraints on language processing: Syntactic priming in Broca's aphasia. *Journal of Cognitive Neuroscience*, *1(3)*, 262-272.

Friederici, A. D. (2004). Processing local transitions versus long-distance syntactic hierarchies. *Trends in Cognitive Science*, *8(6)*, 245-247.

Friederici, A. D., Fiebach, C. J., Schlesewsky, M., Bornkessel, I. D. & von Cramon, D. Y. (2006). Processing linguistic complexity and grammaticality in the left frontal cortex. *Cerebral Cortex, 16(12)*, 1709-1717.

Friederici, A. D., Hahne, A. & von Cramon, D. Y. (1998). First-pass versus second-pass parsing processes in a Wernicke's and a Broca's aphasic: Electrophysiological evidence for a double dissociation. *Brain and Language, 62(3)*, 311-341.

Friederici, A. D., Rüschemeyer, S. A., Hahne, A. & Fiebach, C. J. (2003). The role of left inferior frontal and superior temporal cortex in sentence comprehension: Localizing syntactic and semantic processes. *Cerebral Cortex, 13(2)*, 170-177.

Friedmann, N. A. & Grodzinsky, Y. (1997). Tense and agreement in agrammatic production: Pruning the syntactic tree. *Brain and Language, 56(3)*, 397-425.

Grodzinsky, Y. (2000). The neurology of syntax: Language use without Broca's area. *Behavioral and Brain Science, 23(1)*, 1-71.

Grodzinsky, Y., Piñango, M. M., Zurif, E. & Drai, D. (1999). The critical role of group studies in neuropsychology: Comprehension regularities in Broca's aphasia. *Brain and Language, 67(2)*, 134-147.

Grodzinsky, Y., Wexler, K., Chien, Y. C., Marakovitz, S. & Solomon, J. (1993). The breakdown of binding relations. *Brain and Language, 45(3)*, 396-422.

Haarmann, H. J. & Kolk, H. H. J. (1991). Syntactic priming in Broca's aphasics: Evidence for slow activation. *Aphasiology, 5(3)*, 247-263.

Haarmann, H. J. & Kolk, H. H. J. (1994). On-line sensitivity to subject-verb agreement violations in Broca's aphasics: The role of syntactic complexity and time. *Brain and Language, 46(4)*, 493-516.

Hagège, C. (1974). Les pronoms logophoriques. *Bulletin de la Societe de Linguistique de Paris, 69*, 287-310.

Hagoort, P., Wassenaar, M. & Brown, C. (2003). Real-time semantic compensation in patients with agrammatic comprehension: Electrophysiological evidence for multiple-route plasticity. *Proceedings of the National Academy of Sciences, 100(7)*, 4340-4345.

Hickok, G. & Avrutin, S. (1996). Comprehension of Wh-questions in two Broca's aphasics. *Brain and Language, 52(2)*, 314-327.

Just, M. A., Carpenter, P. A., Keller, T. A., Eddy, W. F. & Thulborn, K. R. (1996). Brain activation modulated by sentence comprehension. *Science, 274(5284)*, 114-116.

Kiran, S. & Thompson, C. K. (2003). Effect of typicality on online category verification of animate category exemplars in aphasia. *Brain and Language, 85(3)*, 441-450.

Kolk, H. H. J. (2000). Multiple route plasticity. *Brain and Language, 71(1)*, 129-131.

Linebarger, M. C., Schwartz, M. F. & Saffran, E. M. (1983). Sensitivity to grammatical structure in so-called agrammatic aphasics. *Cognition, 13(3)*, 361-392.

Love, T., Haist, F., Nicol, J. & Swinney, D. (2006). A functional neuroimaging investigation of the roles of structural complexity and task-demand during auditory sentence processing. *Cortex, 42*, 577-590.

Love, T., Nicol, J., Swinney, D., Hickok, G. & Zurif, E. (1998). The nature of aberrant understanding and processing of pro- forms by brain-damaged populations. *Brain and Language, 65(1)*, 59-62.

Love, T., Swinney, D. & Zurif, E. (2001). Aphasia and the time-course of processing long distance dependencies. *Brain and Language, 79(1)*, 169-170.

Love, T., Swinney, D., Walenski, M. & Zurif, E. (2008). How left inferior frontal cortex participates in syntactic processing: Evidence from aphasia. *Brain and Language, 107(3)*, 203-219.

Lu, C. C., Bates, E., Li, P., Tzeng, O., Hung, D., Tsai, C. H., Lee, S. & Y. M. Chung. (2000). Judgements of grammaticality in aphasia: The special case of Chinese. *Aphasiology, 14(10)*, 1021-1054.

Mauner, G., Fromkin, V. A. & Cornell, T. L. (1993). Comprehension and Acceptability Judgments in Agrammatism: Disruptions in the Syntax of Referential Dependency. *Brain and Language, 45(3)*, 340-370.

Myers, E. B. & Blumstein, S. E. (2005). Selectional restriction and semantic priming effects in normals and Broca's aphasics. *Journal of Neurolinguistics, 18(3)*, 277-296.

Nicol, J. & Swinney, D. (1989). The role of structure in coreference assignment during sentence comprehension T. *Journal of Psycholinguistic Research, 18(1)*, 5-19.

Piñango, M. M. (2000). On the proper generalization for Broca's aphasia comprehension pattern: Why argument movement may not be at the source of the Broca's deficit. *Behavioral and Brain Sciences, 23(1)*, 48-49.

Piñango, M. M. (2002). Cortical reflections of two pronminal relations. In: H. J. Simon, & H. Wiese (Eds.), *Pronouns - grammar and representation* (233-252). Amsterdam: John Benjamins.

Piñango, M. M. (2006). Thematic roles as event structure relations. In: I. Bornkessel, A. D. Friederici, B. Comrie, & M. Schlesewsky (Eds.), *Semantic role universals and argument linking*. Berlin; New York: Mouton de Gruyter.

Prather, P. A., Zurif, E., Love, T. & Brownell, H. (1997). Speed of lexical activation in nonfluent Broca's aphasia and fluent Wernicke's aphasia. *Brain-and-Language, 59(3)*, 391-411.

Röder, B., Stock, O., Neville, H., Bien, S. & Rösler, F. (2002). Brain activation modulated by the comprehension of normal and pseudo-word sentences of different processing demands: A functional magnetic resonance Imaging study. *Neuroimage, 15(4)*, 1003-1014.

Ruigendijk, E., Vasic, N. & Avrutin, S. (2006). Reference assignment: Using language breakdown to choose between theoretical approaches. *Brain and Language, 96(3)*, 302-317.

Sells, P. (1987). Aspects of Logophoricity. *Linguistic-Inquiry, 18(3)*, 445-479.

Shankweiler, D., Crain, S., Gorrell, P. & Tuller, B. (1989). Reception of language in broca's aphasia. *Language and Cognitive Processes, 4(1)*, 1-33.

Swinney, D. & Zurif, E. (1995). Syntactic Processing in Aphasia. *Brain and Language, 50(2)*, 225-239.

Swinney, D., Zurif, E., Prather, P. & Love, T. (1996). Neurological distribution of processing resources underlying language comprehension. *Journal of Cognitive Neuroscience, 8(2)*, 174-184.

Tesak, J. & Dittmann, J. (1991). Telegraphic style in normals and aphasics. *Linguistics, 29(6)*, 1111-1137.

Wulfeck, B., Bates, E. & Capasso, R. (1991). A cross-linguistic study of grammaticality judgments in Broca aphasia. *Brain and Language*, *41(2)*, 311-336.

Zribi-Hertz, A. (1989). Anaphor binding and narrative point of view - English reflexive pronouns in sentence and discourse. *Language*, *65(4)*, 695-727.

Zurif, E., Swinney, D., Prather, P., Solomon, J. & Bushell, C. (1993). An on-line analysis of syntactic processing in Broca's and Wernicke's aphasia. *Brain and Language*, *45(3)*, 448-464.

In: Aphasia: Symptoms, Diagnosis and Treatment
Editors: G. Ibanescu, S. Pescariu

ISBN: 978-1-60741-288-5
© 2009 Nova Science Publishers, Inc.

Chapter V

Synthetic Expressions Do Not Standby[*]

Dieter G. Hillert
University of California, San Diego, USA.

Abstract

Dual-route models and right-hemispheric accounts were suggested to predict comprehension of figurative language in healthy speakers as well as in patients with language disorders. In considering cognitive and neural correlates of recent findings, an alternative model of figurative language comprehension will be discussed. The proposed *Linguistic Analysis-Synthesis* (LAS) model states that "synthetic" expressions do not standby to fill in for "analytical" phrases. The LAS model stipulates only gradual differences between analytical and synthetic lexical computations. Recent neuroimaging evidence supports the view that idiomatic phrases are primarily processed within the left inferior frontal gyrus. It is concluded that the use of frequent expressions produced during chitchats is a much more promising technique to treat fluency disorders in aphasia than the use of idiomatic expressions.

Keywords: Aphasia, Chitchat, Computational Costs, Figurative Language, Fluency Disorder.

Introduction

In recent years, there has been an increasing trend to examine in various healthy and neurological populations the cognitive and neural correlates of synthetic phrases in general and of idiomatic expressions in particular. The expression *rain check*, for instance, may originate to issuing new tickets in form of detachable stubs to baseball fans when a game was rained off. Today, this highly familiar expression is used for negating something in a positive way by postponing an event. Here, we consider an expression as *synthetic* as opposed to *analytic* (propositional), if it combines separate denotative and connotative meanings to form a coherent whole. One reason to focus on synthetic aspects of language processing is that relatively frozen phrases require alternative computations and might therefore recruit neural regions different from analytical computations. Another reason is that synthetic expressions are typically overlearned, automatized strings of lexical units. Thus, here metaphoric phrases (e.g., *The park is the green lung of the city* or *The attorney fought like a lion*) are not considered as synthetic expressions, because they involve lexical creations computed in a non-automatic fashion. A novel metaphor itself is therefore highly analytic, since lexical combinations are constructed in a completely new fashion. The question arises therefore whether certain synthetic elements are spared in aphasic patients. A language treatment program based on specific types of synthetic expressions might be an extremely valuable instrument to enhance fluency and possibly the production of meaningful phrases in aphasic patients.

One excellent category of synthetic elements seem to be discourse markers used during chitchats (e.g., *hi, how are you, enjoy your meal, you know, let's see, have a nice day*). They are the most frequent lexical items and phrases in spontaneous speech (Moon, 1998). In contrast, Jackendoff (1995) notes that the number of idioms as well as of other synthetic entries (e.g., names, titles, poems) have at least the same order of magnitude as the number of single words. Strässler (1982) counted an idiomatic expression every 4.5 min of text, which seems to be a much lower rate than anticipated for discourse markers. Even Van Lancker-Sidtis & Rallona's (2004) analysis of Billy Wilder's screenplay *Some like it hot* revealed that idioms (145) were produced much less than speech formula (377). The discrepancy between these numbers is conservative, since a screenplay may include a larger amount of synthetic expressions than "standard" spontaneous speech. Let us look more closely at the cognitive and neural correlates of synthetic expressions and their potential for aphasic treatment programs.

Computational Aspects of Synthetic Language

Before turning in details to the computational aspects of synthetic expressions, it is worthwhile to have a closer look at their structural characteristics. Speakers are typically not aware of the etymology of a synthetic expression, but somehow these expressions became fossilized. For instance, an unfamiliar idiomatic phrase is peculiar to itself as such that we understand the meaning of each word of the phrase as well as the entire grammatical structure without being able to understand the implicit meaning it carries. However, in case of familiar idiomatic phrases, we typically know how to use these synthetic expressions in a specific pragmatic context. The conveyed meaning of those expressions is often colorful and imaginary to express subjective values and intentions. In contrast to short synthetic forms, longer expression such as *to let the cat out of the bag* might refer to a literal event, although it

* Supported by the "Japan Society for the Promotion of Science" (FY2007 JSPS). I am grateful to Professor Yoko Nakano and the Faculty of Humanities and Economics at Kochi University for their hospitality. Send correspondence to dhillert@ucsd.edu.

may be obviously less frequently used than the synthetic reading. Truly synthetic is the expression *It is raining cats and dogs,* because it can only be realized in our imagination or via animation that cats and dogs fall from the sky such as rain drops.

Different computational models have been proposed to predict how people process idiomatic expressions. Early models postulated a passive lexical storage device. For instance, Bobrow & Bell (1973) postulated a separate idiom list, which listeners would recruit when the literal interpretation fails; Swinney & Cutler (1979) suggested that idioms are stored as morphologically complex words in the mental lexicon, and both figurative and literal meanings would be accessed in parallel before context selects the appropriate reading. In contrast, Gibbs' (1980) "direct access hypothesis" implies that the figurative meaning of an idiom will be accessed directly without activating literal meanings at all. Again, Cacciari & Tabossi's (1988) "configuration hypothesis" predicts that the figurative meaning of an idiomatic expression will be accessed at the idiom key, that is, after the listener encountered a specific lexical configuration.

Gibbs, Nayak, & Cutting (1989) introduced the "decomposition hypothesis" to examine whether access to the synthetic reading involves analytical or (de)compositional computations. The idiom *pop the question,* for instance, was considered to be a "normal decomposable" idiom as each part contributes to the overall synthetic meaning (*pop*: make; *the question*: a marriage proposal). The idiom *carry a torch* was considered as an "abnormal decomposable" idiom, since only one element of the expression refers to a figurative concept (*torch*: warm feelings). Finally, in a "non-decomposable" idiom no single element seems to contribute to the figurative reading (e.g., *chew the fat*). That subjects' latencies to (de)composable (normal and abnormal) idioms were shorter than to their literal counterparts (e.g., *ask the question* or *light the torch*) was regarded as evidence in favor of a literal-independent process model. However, this conclusion is truly biased, because it is not difficult to create a scenario that leads to the opposite interpretation. For instance, the process of judging a single lexical unit may occur faster than judging a lexical phrase. Linguistic judgments involve a wrap-up effect and it seems to be plausible that the wrap-up effect for fixed meanings is faster than for (de)compositional meanings. In both cases, however, the literal meaning may have been accessed in an automatic fashion. This interpretation is supported by the finding that latencies for "non-decomposable" phrases were significantly slower than for the literal control phrases. Automatically activated literal meanings may need to be inhibited in case of non-decomposable strings. This effect may have led to longer latencies compared to non-figuratively interpretable literal phrases.

Giora's (1997) theoretically driven approach emphasizes the interplay between the saliency of an expression and the strength of the biasing sentence context. Thus, there is no unique mechanism for idiom comprehension, but it is a combination of different factors that determines how fast people understand a particular synthetic expression. Finally, Titone & Connine's (1999) "hybrid model" predicts that initially both the figurative as well as the literal meaning of a decomposable or non-decomposable phrase will be activated. However, similar to Gibbs et al.'s (1989) results, their eye-tracking study indicates that it takes longer to integrate non-decomposable idioms than decomposable ones. Titone & Connine assume therefore that non-decomposable idiomatic meanings are retrieved in one step, while access to the meaning of decomposable idioms occurs much like an inferential procedure.

These different models and hypotheses illustrate that there are multiple process mechanism associated with comprehension of synthetic expressions. It is difficult to compare data, if the experimental parameters differ largely in terms of input modality, task condition, mode of processing, etc. (Hillert & Swinney, 2000). Most of all, the psycholinguistic work addresses a large range of different synthetic expressions. The variability in stimulus presentation makes it quite difficult or impossible to construct a unitary model of synthetic language processing based on psycholinguistic data. In addition, some neuropsychological models have been also proposed to predict the neural correlates of different types of figurative meanings.

Neural Correlates of Synthetic Language

In the middle of 19th century, the rise of cognitive neuropsychology, researchers already noted that aphasic patients have less difficulty to produce common phrases than propositional speech. Jackson (1878), for instance, observed consistently preserved speech forms carrying emotional aspects, but a disorder for intellectual-propositional speech; Marie (1925) emphasized the dissociation between voluntary and automatic speech; Head (1926), who introduced the concept of "asymbolism", observed that aphasic patients seem to rely on non-propositional speech, and Pick (1931) considered automatic speech as being spared in aphasia. Again, in the second half of the 20th century many aphasiologists discussed the distinction between propositional and non-propositional speech in patients with chronic aphasia (e.g., Luria, 1947; Goldstein, 1948; Alajouanine, 1956; Goodglass & Mayer, 1958; Luria, 1966; see for a review Van Lancker-Sidtis, 2006). Language production in chronic aphasic patients' seems to circumscribe basic "chitchatting" abilities, which essentially include overlearned lexical sequences such as common phrases, rhymes, lyrics, counting fixed sequences (e.g., numbers or time sequences).

However, in the past it has been claimed that processing figurative language is lateralized in the right hemisphere. This right-hemisphere hypothesis based on behavioral data collected from patients with unilateral lesions (e.g., Winner & Gardner, 1977; Brownell, Potter, Michelow, & Gardner, 1984; Van Lancker & Kempler, 1987; Weylman, Brownell, Roman, & Gardner, 1989; Huber, 1990; Joanette, Goulet, & Hannequin, 1990; Burgess & Chiarello, 1996). But these studies imply serious methodological problems. First, the large variety of figurative stimuli tested does not allow a direct comparison between these different datasets. Second, often the task condition requires matching a selected word or phrase to a target picture illustrating the appropriate figurative and/or literal meaning. These verbal-pictorial matching tasks are quite artificial, since neither patients' pre-onset usage of specific figurative expressions were controlled nor the impact of a particular lesion site. For instance, it has been reported that the right cerebral cortex plays a particular role in visuospatial processing (Jordan & Hillis, 2005) or is in charge of suppressing automatic activations of literal meanings. Third, lesion studies with aphasic patients indicate that "figurative" processing is not necessarily a domain of the right cortex. In using a sentence-to-picture/word task, left-hemispheric patients seemed to have had particular difficulties with understanding metaphoric and/or idiomatic expressions (e.g., Giora, Zaidel, Soroker, Batori, & Kasher,

2000; Papagno, Tabossi, Colombo, & Zampetti, 2004; Cacciari, Reati, Colombo, Padovani, Rizzo, & Papagno, 2006). Other studies, however, point to the opposite interpretation as such that "non-propositional" language seems to be relatively less impaired in aphasia in contrast to propositional language (e.g., Whitaker, 1976; Nakagawa, Tanabe, Ikeda, Kazui, Ito, Inoue, Hatakenaka, Atakenaka, Sawada, Ikeda, & Shiraishi, 1993; Lum & Ellis, 1994; Van Lancker & Bella, 1996). Moreover, several lesion studies indicate no cortex-specific role for synthetic expressions (e.g., Tompkins, Boada, & McGarry, 1992; Chobor & Schweiger, 1998; Gagnon, Goulet, Giroux, & Joanette, 2003; Hillert, 2004). In sum, the outcome of these different lesion studies indicates that lesion etiology, task condition, type of stimulus material (e.g., the use of a wide range of synthetic expressions) and control group (e.g., comparison between aphasic patients and non-age matched healthy controls) are confounding factors that do not permit to draw *general* conclusions about the neural correlates of synthetic expressions. Overall, however, it appears that the speech of aphasic patients during early post-onset treatment relies on discourse markers or overlearned sequences (e.g., Code, 1982; Graves & Landis, 1985; Blanken, 1991). Other synthetic expressions such as idoms or metaphors seem not to be particularly preserved in aphasia (but see Van Lancker-Sidtis, 2001).

Neuroimaging studies conducted mostly with healthy controls revealed also conflicting results. For instance, Bottini, Corcoran, Sterzi, Paulesu, Schenone, Scarpa, Frackowiak, & Frith's (1994) PET study noted greater right-sided cortical activity in the inferior frontal gyrus (IFG) and the posterior temporal lobe for metaphors as compared to literal meanings. Similar, Ahrens, Liu, Lee, C.Y., Gong, Fang, & Hsu (2007) reported in their fMRI study particular activity in the right cerebral cortex for conventional and novel metaphors. Oliveri, Romero, & Papagno (2004), who used repetitive transcranial magnetic stimulation (rTMS), found that left temporal rTMS disrupted participants' performance in a sentence-to-picture matching task. Because this effect was not obtained after rTMS over the right cortex, it was concluded that the left temporal lobe plays a particular role in comprehension of idiomatic and literal language. Moreover, some fMRI studies with healthy speakers revealed that the classical language areas seem to be involved in idiom comprehension (e.g., Lee & Dapretto, 2006; Hillert & Buracas, 2009), but others reported bilateral activities (e.g., Lauro, Tettamanti, & Cappa, 2008; Zempleni, Haverkort, Renken, & Stowe, 2007).

In light of these new data, it is difficult to maintain a right-hemisphere account for common idiomatic expressions. The right-cerebral cortex seem to be more involved in processing or constructing novel meanings as it is required for metaphor comprehension (cf. Rapp, Leube, Erb, Grodd, & Kircher, 2007). The fundamental question arises whether the intensity of neural activity is associated with different meaning types. It appears that the factor "cognitive complexity" is a more reliable predictor for human brain mapping than subtypes of lexical or phrasal meanings. What kind of information will be processed in which cortical region, seems to be largely dependent on the computational costs associated with a certain task condition. Common synthetic expressions seem to be a domain of the classical language areas, since they do not imply additional computational costs as compared to non-figurative speech. Novel information, including metaphoric meanings, engages broader cortical areas including regions of the right hemisphere. Which brain areas are involved in linguistic processing seems to be exclusively a matter of the computational resource requirements. In the following a computational model of synthetic expressions will be briefly discussed that emphasizes relevant interactions between different types of computations.

The Linguistic Analysis-Synthesis Model

The mainstream of research such as dual route models states that synthetic phrases are processed qualitatively different than analytical word combinations. Empirical evidence, as discussed before, indicates however that the type of computations involved in comprehension of synthetic language is largely dependent on several cognitive and linguistic factors. *Synthetic expressions do not standby to fill in for lexical gaps.* They carry as any other lexical entry specific and irreplaceable specific meanings. "Approximate synonymy" applies not only to analytical but also to synthetic language.

Here we discuss the *Linguistic Analysis-Synthesis* (LAS) model that stipulates only gradual differences between analytical and synthetic computations. During sentence processing strings of lexical entries are sequentially combined in a bottom-up fashion, while simultaneously top-down information facilitates or determines the comprehension process (Hillert & Ackerman, 2002). For instance, listeners combine lexical entries, which are already perceived, with incoming linguistic information. Lexical strings are composed out of single phonemes and syntactic units are merged to generate higher-order lexical phrases. Pragmatic cues and linguistic probabilities secure a constant interaction between input stream and top-down information. Figure 1 illustrates some analytical and synthetic computations involved in online (real-time) comprehension of a common idiomatic expression. After the initial time modifier *It's time* and after the verb phrase (VP) *to let* and the second NP *the cat,* the listener perceives the preposition *out.* Depending on context cues and subjective familiarity of a synthetic reading, the listener may revise her/his initial analytical parse.

It may be in the grammatical vicinity of *cat out of* (the idiom key) that the listener uses top-down information to activate the synthetic reading. However, it is to assume that this top-down process will interfere within the ongoing analytical bottom-up process. Psycholinguistic findings indicate that the analytical bottom-up process continues simultaneously or will be actively inhibited, depending on the strength of contextual information. The length of the "idiom onset" can be considered as the onset cue for a synthetic entry. On encountering the idiom key, the parser needs to track back previous lexical input, kept in a short-term buffer, to revise its initial analytical parse. It is obvious that the interaction between analytical and synthetic processes involves higher computational costs than unambiguous speech. This account is supported by the above mentioned fMRI data that indicate the involvement of the left IFG (particularly Broca's area and vicinity) in idiom comprehension. In general, cortical activity of Broca's area in comparison to left temporal structures has been taken as evidence for an increase in cognitive resource demand reflected in higher computational costs (e.g., Kaan & Swaab, 2002; Mason, Just, Keller and Carpenter, 2003; Hillert, 2008). Therefore, the LAS model does not predict that idiomatic expressions are good candidates for treating fluency disorders in aphasia.

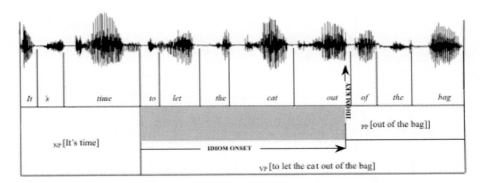

Figure 1. Online comprehension of an idiomatic expression (see text).

Conclusion

The cognitive and neural correlates of synthetic expressions typically require more computational resources than unambiguous propositional language. Only a certain subset of synthetic expressions appears adequate for treating fluency disorders in aphasia. Doubtless, an individually customized treatment strategy may be advantageous as such that data are available about the patient's pre-onset language abilities. Otherwise, it may be important to consider subject-specific knowledge. For instance, a stock broker may have used certain financial terms more frequently, and using these terms in therapy may help the broker's ability to re-activate particular lexical semantic fields. As far as synthetic language is concerned, lexical elements and phrases used during chitchats or small talks seemed to be the best candidates for initiating lexical or linguistic processing. Discourse markers are mainly used only for conversational reasons and involve minimal computational costs. This is the reason that there are typically the most promising lexical units to facilitate recovering linguistic computations.

References

Ahrens, K., Liu, H. L., Lee, C. Y., Gong, S. P., Fang, S. Y. & Hsu, Y. Y. (2007). Functional MRI of conventional and anomalous metaphors in Mandarin Chinese. *Brain and Language, 100(2)*, 163-171.

Alajouanine, T. (1956) Verbal realization in aphasia. *Brain, 79,* 1-28.

Blanken, G. (1991). The functional basis of speech automatisms (recurring utterances). *Aphasiology, 5,* 103-127.

Bobrow, S. A. & Bell, S. M. (1973). On catching on to idiomatic expressions. *Memory & Cognition, 1(3),* 343-346.

Bottini, G., Corcoran, R., Sterzi, R., Paulesu, E., Schenone, P., Scarpa, P., Frackowiak, R. S. & Frith, C. D. (1994). The role of the right hemisphere in the interpretation of figurative aspects of language. A positron emission tomography activation study. *Brain, 117(6),* 1241-1253.

Brownell, H. H., Potter, H. H., Michelow, D. & Gardner, H. (1984). Sensitivity to lexical denotation and connotation in brain-damaged patients: a double dissociation? *Brain and Language, 29*, 310-321.

Burgess, C. & Chiarello, C. (1996). Neurocognitive mechanisms underlying metaphor comprehension and other figurative language. *Metaphor and Symbolic Activity, 11*, 67-84.

Cacciari, C. & Tabossi, P. (1988). The comprehension of idioms. *Journal of Memory and Language, 27*, 668-683.

Cacciari, C., Reati, F., Colombo, M. R., Padovani, R, Rizzo, S. & Papagno, C. (2006). The comprehension of ambiguous idioms in aphasic patients. *Neuropsychologia, 44(8)*, 1305-14.

Chobor, K. & Schweiger, A. (1998). Processing of lexical ambiguity in patients with traumatic brain injury. *Journal of Neurolinguistics, 11*, 119-136.

Code, C. (1982). Neurolinguistic analysis of recurrent utterance in aphasia. *Cortex, 18*, 141-152.

Gagnon, L., Goulet, P., Giroux, F. & Joanette, Y. (2003). Processing of metaphoric and non-metaphoric alternative meanings of words and right- and left- hemispheric lesion. *Brain and Language, 87*, 217-226.

Gibbs, & O'Brien, J. (1990). Idioms and mental imagery: the metaphorical motivation for idiom meaning. *Cognition, 36*, 35-68.

Gibbs, R. (1980). Spilling the beans on understanding and memory for idioms in conversation. *Memory and Cognition*, 8, 149-56.

Gibbs, R. W., Nayak, N. P. & Cutting, C. (1989). How to kick the bucket and not decompose: Analyzability and idiom processing. *Journal of Memory and Language, 28*, 576–593.

Giora, R. (1997). Understanding figurative language: The graded salience hypothesis. *Cognitive Linguistics, 7(1)*, 183-206.

Giora, R., Zaidel, E., Soroker, N., Batori, G. & Kasher, A. (2000). Differential effect of right- and left hemisphere damage on understanding sarcasm and metaphor. *Metaphor and Symbolic Activity, 15*, 63.

Goldstein, K. (1948). *Language and language disturbance*. New York: Grune & Stratton.

Goodglass, H. & Mayer, J. (1958). Agrammatism in aphasia. *Journal of Speech and Hearing Disorders, 23*, 99-111.

Graves, R. & Landis, T. (1985). Hemispheric control of speech expression in aphasia. *Archives of Neurology, 42*, 249-251.

Head, H. (1926). Aphasia and kindred disorders of speech. (repr.) *Neurosurgery*, 1998, *42(4)*, 944-948.

Hillert, D. & Ackerman, F. (2002). Accessing and parsing phrasal predicates. In: N. Dehé, R. Jackendoff, A. McIntryre, & S. Urban (Eds.), *Verb-Particle Explorations*. Berlin: Mouton de Gruyter.

Hillert, D. G. & Buracas, G. T. (2009). The neural substrates of spoken idiom comprehension. *Language and Cognitive Processes*. (in press)

Hillert, D. G. & Swinney, D. A. (2000). The processing of fixed expressions during sentence comprehension. In: A. Cienki, B. J. Luka, B. J. & M. B. Smith (Eds.), *Conceptual structure, discourse, and language*. Stanford: CSLI.

Hillert, D. G. (2004). Spared access to idiomatic and literal meanings: a single-case approach. *Brain and Language, 89(1)*, 207-215.

Hillert, D. G. (2008). On idioms: Cornerstones for a neurological model of language processing. *Journal of Cognitive Science 9 (2)*, 193-233.

Huber, W. (1990). Text comprehension and production in aphasia: Analysis in terms of micro- and macroprocessing. In: Y. Joanette, & H. H. Brownell (Eds.), *Discourse ability and brain damage: Theoretical and empirical perspectives*. New York: Springer Press.

Jackendoff, R. (1995). The boundaries of the lexicon. In: M. Everaert, E. J. van der Linden, A. Schenk, & R. Schreuder, (Eds.), *Idioms, structural and psychological perspectives*. Hillsdale: LEA.

Jackson, J. H. (1878). On affections of speech from disease of the brain. *Brain, 1*, 304-330.

Joanette, Y., Goulet, P. & Hannequin, D. (1990). *Right hemisphere and verbal communication*. Springer Press.

Jordan, L. C. & Hillis, A. E. (2005). Aphasia and right hemisphere syndromes in stroke. *Current Neurology and Neuroscience Reports, 5*, 458-464.

Kaan, E. & Swaab, T. Y. (2002). The brain circuitry of syntactic comprehension. *Trends in Cognitive Science, 6*, 350-356.

Lauro, L. J. R., Tettamanti, M., Cappa, S. F. & Papagno, C. (2008). Idiom comprehension: A prefrontal task? *Cerebral Cortex, 18*, 162-170.

Lee, S. S. & Dapretto, M. (2006). Metaphorical vs. literal word meanings: fMRI evidence against a selective role of the right hemisphere. *Neuroimage, 29(2)*, 536-544.

Lum, C. C. & Ellis, A. W. (1994). Is 'non-propositional' speech preserved in aphasia? *Brain and Language, 46*, 368-391.

Luria, A. R. (1947). *Traumatic Aphasia: Its Syndromes, Psychopathology and Treatment*. Moscow: Academy of Medical Sciences.

Luria, A. R. (1966). *Higher Cortical Functions in Man*. New York: Basic.

Mason, R. A., Just, M. A., Keller, T. A. & Carpenter, P. A. (2003). Ambiguity in the brain: what brain imaging reveals about the processing of syntactically implicit sentences. *Journal of Experimental Psychology: Learning, Memory, & Cognition, 29(6)*, 1319-1338.

Moon, R. E. (1998). Frequencies and forms of phrasal lexemes in English. In: A. P. Cowie (ed.) *Phraseology*. Oxford: Clarenden Press.

Nakagawa, Y., Tanabe, H., Ikeda, M., Kazui, H., Ito, K., Inoue, N., Hatakenaka, Y., Atakenaka, Y., Sawada, T., Ikeda, H. & Shiraishi, J. (1993). Completion phenomenon in transcortical sensory aphasia. *Behavioural Neurology, 6*, 135-142.

Oliveri, M., Romero, L. & Papagno, C. (2004). Left but not right temporal involvement in opaque idiom comprehension: a repetitive transcranial magnetic stimulation study. *Journal of Cognitive Neuroscience, 16*, 848-855.

Papagno, C., Tabossi, P., Colombo, M. R. & Zampetti, P. (2004). Idiom comprehension in aphasic patients. *Brain and Language, 89*, 226-234.

Pick, A. (1931). *Aphasia*. Springfield: Thomas.

Rapp, A. M., Leube, D. T., Erb, M., Grodd, W. & Kircher, T. T. (2007). Laterality in metaphor processing: lack of evidence from functional magnetic resonance imaging for the right hemisphere theory. *Brain and Language, 100(2)*, 142-149.

Swinney, D. & Cutler, A. (1979). The access and processing of idiomatic expressions. *Journal of Verbal Learning and Verbal Behavior*, *18*, 523-534.

Titone, D. & Connine, C. (1999). On the compositional and noncompositional nature of idiomatic expressions. *Journal of Pragmatics*, *31*, 1655-1674.

Tompkins, C. A., Boada, R. & McGarry, K. (1992). The access and processing of familiar idioms by brain damaged and normally aging adults. *Journal of Speech and Hearing Research*, *35*, 626-637.

Van Lancker Sidtis (2006). Where in the Brain Is Nonliteral Language? *Metaphor and Symbol*, *21(4)*, 213-244.

Van Lancker, D. & Bella, R. (1996). The relative roles of repetition and sentence completion tasks in revealing superior speech abilities in patients with nonfluent aphasia. *Journal of the International Neuropsychological Society*, *2*, 6.

Van Lancker, D. & Kempler, D. (1987). Comprehension of familiar phrases by left- but not by right-hemisphere damaged patients. *Brain and Language*, *32*, 265-277.

Van Lancker-Sidtis, D. & Rallon, G. (2004).Tracking the incidence of formulaic expressions in everyday speech: Methods for classification and verification. *Language and Communication*, *24*, 207-240.

Van Lancker-Sidtis, D. (2001). Preserved formulaic expressions in a case of transcortical sensory aphasia compared to incidence in normal everyday speech. *Brain and Language*, *79(1)*, 38-41.

Weylman, S. T., Brownell, H. H., Roman, M. & Gardner, H. (1989). Appreciation of indirect request by left- and right-brain damaged patients: The effects of verbal context and conventionality of wording. *Brain and Language*, *36*, 580-591.

Whitaker, H. A. (1976). A case of isolation of the speech functions. In: H. Whitaker, & H. A. Whitaker (eds.) *Studies in Neurolinguistics*, Vol 2. London: Academic Press.

Winner, E. & Gardner, H. (1977). The comprehension of metaphor in brain-damaged patients. *Brain*, *100*, 719-727.

Zemplenia, M. Z., Haverkortd, M., Renkenb, R. & Stowe, L. A. (2007). Evidence for bilateral involvement in idiom comprehension: An fMRI study. *Neuroimage*, *34(3)*, 1280-1291.

In: Aphasia: Symptoms, Diagnosis and Treatment   ISBN: 978-1-60741-288-5
Editors: G. Ibanescu, S. Pescariu   © 2009 Nova Science Publishers, Inc.

Chapter VI

Lateralizing Value of Postictal Perseveration in Temporal Lobe Epilepsy

Andras Fogarasi[*]

Epilepsy Center, National Institute of Psychiatry and Neurology, Budapest, Hungary.
Epilepsy Center, Bethesda Children's Hospital, Budapest, Hungary.

Abstract

Purpose

To describe clinical characteristics and lateralizing value of postictal perseveration (repetitive verbal behavior) in patients with temporal lobe epilepsy (TLE). Other postictal language disorders (aphasia, paraphasia) are well-described signs in TLE; however, postictal perseveration has not been systematically analyzed so far.

Methods

One hundred and ninety-three videotaped seizures of 55 consecutive patients with refractory TLE and postoperatively seizure-free outcome were analyzed. Postictal perseveration was monitored.

Results

Perseveration was observed during the postictal period in 18 (9%) of the 193 seizures. The phenomenon occurred more frequently after left-sided seizures (16 left-sided and two right-sided; p=0.002). Neither age at epilepsy onset, age at monitoring,

---

[*] Corresponding author: András Fogarasi, MD, PhD, Epilepsy Center, Bethesda Children's Hospital, H-1146-Budapest, Bethesda Street 3, Hungary. Fax: +36-1-3649070; Email: fogarasi@bethesda.hu

duration of epilepsy nor gender were significantly different between patients with and without postictal perseveration.

Conclusion

Postictal perseveration is a rare phenomenon in TLE but lateralizes the seizure onset zone to the left hemisphere. Our observation can help the presurgical evaluation of TLE because verbal perseveration frequently occurs spontaneously, even in seizures without appropriate postictal language testing.

Key words: Temporal lobe epilepsy, lateralizing signs, aphasia, perseveration.

Introduction

Postictal aphasia and dysphasia are well-described phenomena in temporal lobe epilepsy (TLE) lateralizing the seizure onset zone to the dominant hemisphere (Gabr et al., 1989). Assessing these phenomena usually requires proper testing right after the end of a seizure. In many cases, however, postictal testing is not available. In these situations, a spontaneous form of aphasia, i.e., postictal perseveration (PP) (Basso, 2004) could be a reasonably used lateralizing sign. Because no clinical study has so far assessed PP, the aim of our study was to systematically evaluate the frequency, characteristics and lateralizing value of PP in patients with TLE.

Patients and Methods

We analyzed archived seizures of all patients between 1992 and 2005 who underwent presurgical evaluation at the National Institute of Psychiatry and Neurology and the Bethesda Children's Hospital (both in Budapest, Hungary) and became seizure-free after temporal lobe resection (with a postoperative follow-up of minimum one year). Age at onset of epilepsy ranged between 10 months and 35 years (mean 13.8 ± 8.5 years), and age at video-EEG monitoring was 9 to 49 (mean 30.4 ± 10.1) years. Postoperative histology showed hippocampal sclerosis (36), tumor (10), and focal cortical dysplasia (in nine patients). Each patient typically had two to seven (mean 3.7) archived seizures.

Time-labeled video recordings of 205 seizures from 55 patients (30 with left-sided TLE) were reviewed by an investigator (A.F.) blinded to the patients' clinical and EEG data as well as site of operation. From this pool, 193 seizure records (24 with secondarily generalization) contained at least two minutes of analyzable postictal state. In 11 cases, patients fell asleep right after seizure, and an additional seizure occurred right after the end of the ictal period. Each of these 193 seizures (105 [54%] left-sided) was analyzed with regard to the presence and characteristics of any PP.

Postictal perseveration was defined as any repetitive verbal behavior including stereotypy or echolalia (Hudson, 1968; Christman et al., 2004). This could be repetition of a syllable, word, neologism or even a short sentence (Basso, 2004; Sandson and Albert, 1984).

Postictal perseveration rarely was reactive to the testing task (e.g., echolalia of the question); rather, it was independent of it. The testing person could not interrupt this behavior by additional questions or tasks.

Beside PP assessment, each seizure was classified by a semiological seizure classification (Luders et al., 1998). Data were analyzed for univariate analyses, using binomial and Fisher's exact tests. The Mann-Whitney test was used to check any association between the presence of PP and age at monitoring, age at onset as well as duration of epilepsy of patients. Two-tailed error probabilities lower than $p<0.05$ were considered to be significant. All statistical analyses were carried out with the SPSS 11.5 statistical package for WINDOWS (SPSS Inc., Chicago).

Results

Postictal perseveration was observed in 18 (9%) seizures. It contained different—always comprehendible but usually inadequate—simple verbal expressions such as "I don't know", "Yes", "No", "Good", "Nothing", "Why?", "All right", etc. More complicated PPs were rare; the most complex was "What should I say?" Four of these 18 PPs were answers to the testing questions while the others were independent of postictal testing. All patients with postictal speech automatisms were right-handed.

Postictal perseveration occurred more frequently after left-sided seizures (16 left-sided and two right-sided; $p=0.002$). Neither age at epilepsy onset, age at monitoring, duration of epilepsy nor gender were significantly different between patients with and without PA. Seizures with PPs contained mostly automotor seizure components, but tonic and clonic components also occurred. Perseveration happened exclusively during the postictal period and never started ictally. From the 18 seizures with PP, only 10 attacks (56%) also contained postictal dysphasia.

Discussion

Our study using retrospective semiology data of 193 seizures showed that PP is a relatively infrequent phenomenon in TLE but lateralizes the seizure onset zone in the left hemisphere. Other postictal language disorders (aphasia, paraphasia) are well-known left-sided lateralizing signs in TLE; however, PP has not been systematically analyzed so far. According to neuropsychological studies, perseveration is a frequent phenomenon in patients with aphasia (Yamadori, 1981; Santo Pietro and Rigrodsky, 1986; Helm-Estabrooks et al., 1998). One study assessed the frequency of perseveration in 50 aphasic patients due to left-sided brain damage (Basso, 2004). Twenty of them (40%) showed two or more instances of perseveration during neuropsychological language tasks. Another study observed perseverations in 14/148 (9%) patients during an intracarotid amobarbital test (Kurthen et al., 1992). Verbal perseveration occurred exclusively at the start of left-sided amobarbital injection. Language testing during the Wada test proved left hemispheric speech dominance in all of these cases. These data support the hypothesis that perseveration is a right hemispheric continuation of a speech motor program previously initiated by the left hemisphere (Kurthen et al., 1992). We think that the left hemispheric dominance of PP can be explained by a similar mechanism due to the postictal exhaustion of the dominant hemisphere. It is important to note that most seizures with PP contained no postictal dysphasia, emphasizing the possible complementary role of PP in lateralizing the seizure onset zone.

Our results can help the presurgical evaluation of patients with TLE because perseveration frequently occurs spontaneously even in seizures without appropriate postictal language testing.

Acknowledgment

The study was supported by the Bolyai Scholarship of the Hungarian Academy of Sciences.

References

Basso, A. (2004). Perseveration or the Tower of Babel. *Semin Speech Lang*, *25*, 375-389.

Christman, S. S., Boutsen, F. R. & Buckingham, H. W. (2004). Perseveration and other repetitive verbal behaviors: functional dissociations. *Semin Speech Lang*, *25*, 295-308.

Gabr, M., Luders, H., Dinner, D., Morris, H. & Wyllie, E. (1989). Speech manifestations in lateralization of temporal lobe seizures. *Ann Neurol.*, *25*, 82-87.

Helm-Estabrooks, N., Ramage, A., Bayles, K. A. & Cruz, R. (1998). Perseverative behavior in fluent and non-fluent aphasic adults. *Aphasiology*, *12*, 689-698.

Hudson, A. J. (1968). Perseveration. *Brain*, *91*, 571-582.

Kurthen, M., Linke, D. B., Elger, C. E. & Schramm, J. (1992). Linguistic perseveration in dominant-side intracarotid amobarbital tests. *Cortex*, *28*, 209-219.

Luders, H., Acharya, J., Baumgartner, C., Benbadis, S., Bleasel, A., Burgess, R., Dinner, D. S., Ebner, A., Foldvary, N., Geller, E., Hamer, H., Holthausen, H., Kotagal, P., Morris, H., Meencke, H. J., Noachtar, S., Rosenow, F., Sakamoto, A., Steinhoff, B. J., Tuxhorn, I. & Wyllie, E. (1998). Semiological seizure classification. *Epilepsia*, *39*, 1006-1013.

Sandson, J. & Albert, M. L. (1984). Varieties of perseveration. *Neuropsychologia*, *22*, 715-732.

Santo Pietro, M. J. & Rigrodsky, S. (1986). Patterns of oral-verbal perseveration in adult aphasics. *Brain Lang*, *19*, 1-17.

Yamadori, A. (1981). Verbal perseveration in aphasia. *Neuropsychologia*, *19*, 591-594.

In: Aphasia: Symptoms, Diagnosis and Treatment
Editors: G. Ibanescu, S. Pescariu

ISBN: 978-1-60741-288-5
© 2009 Nova Science Publishers, Inc.

Chapter VII

Assessment and Treatment of Bilingual Aphasia and Bilingual Anomia

[1]Patricia M. Roberts and [2]Swathi Kiran
[1]Audiology and Speech-Language Pathology Program, University of Ottawa,
Ottawa, Ontario, Canada).
[2]Department of Communication Sciences and Disorders,
University of Texas at Austin, Austin, Texas, USA

Introduction

This chapter will present a general framework for looking at bilingual aphasia and will review issues relevant to the assessment and treatment of anomia in bilingual aphasic adults. Anomia is the most universal symptom in aphasia, and one which patients find frustrating. It is also one of the best studied areas in aphasia, drawing on a large body of knowledge about lexical models, lexical access, and the naming process in non-aphasic adults.

This chapter begins by defining some of the key terminology. The bulk of the chapter is devoted to a discussion of current assessment methods, especially assessment of naming impairments, and a review of studies on the rehabilitation of bilingual aphasia, with a particular focus on the assessment and treatment of naming (or word-finding) The chapter closes with a commentary on various methodological issues and steps to foster more rapid progress in the field of bilingual aphasia.

Some Definitions

Aphasia: For this chapter, "aphasia" refers only to the language impairment caused by strokes, since this is the area that has been most studied. The progressive language loss that is part of most dementias is, many authors and clinicians feel, a different disorder.

Bilingual aphasia: The term "bilingual aphasia" is generally used as a shorthand for "aphasia occurring in bilingual speaker-hearers". Although some studies of trilinguals and multilinguals are now appearing (e.g., de Bot, 2004; Goral, Levy, Obler, and Cohen, 2006; Goral and Obler, in press; Lemhöfer, Dijkstra, and Michel, 2004), we do not yet know if there are differences between bilingual and multilingual speakers with aphasia (for example, in their symptoms, prognosis, or treatment outcomes). So, for now, the term "bilingual aphasia" generally refers to multilinguals as well as to bilinguals.

Bilingualism: In this chapter, the term "bilingual" is used to describe people with a range of levels of knowledge of a second language. It is not restricted to the so-called "perfect mastery" of two languages, since it is now clear that this level may be unattainable, for a variety of reasons (Butler and Hakuta, 2006; Christophersen, 1999; Hyltenstam, 1992), including the influences, in both directions, between each language spoken (e.g., Dijkstra, del Prado, Fermin, Schulpen, Schreuder, and Baayen, 2005; Edwards, 2006; Levey, 2004; Pavlenko, 2000; Pavlenko and Jarvis, 2002; Van Hell and Dijkstra, 2002; Van Wijnendaele and Brysbaert, 2002).

We view each individual's level of bilingualism (LOB) not as a unitary thing, but as something that varies across modalities, along a continuum of proficiency within each modality. As do many other authors, we see bilingualism as multidimensional, with each individual at some level of expertise in auditory comprehension, verbal expression, reading, and writing. An overall rating of proficiency is not very informative and we should not expect high correlations between overall ratings and performance on specific tasks. Readers with expertise in aphasia recognize these modalities as part of the grid used in aphasia assessments and in planning treatment, since each modality may be differentially affected by the aphasia. It is relatively recent for these four modalities to serve as a framework for describing a bilingual speaker's level of proficiency in each language.

As Grosjean (1989) and others have said: the bilingual speaker is unlike a native speaker of either language. These two facts (bidirectional influence between languages and competency being along modality-specific continua) present problems for the assessment and treatment of aphasia, as this chapter will show.

Importance of Bilingual Aphasia

As noted by previous authors, the high incidence of bilingualism in many parts of the world (e.g., Fabbro, 2001; Harris, 1992; Paradis, 1995) and the universal presence of strokes combine to produce large numbers of bilingual adults with aphasia (Paradis, 2001). There is a professional obligation to understand the disorder, to develop treatment methods and to assess their efficacy. In 1998, Roberts found that the existing literature was "sparse in relation to the clinical importance of understanding bilingual aphasia in order to assist bilingual adults recovering from and living with their aphasia" (Roberts, 1998b, p. 145). Since 1998, there has been an increase in the number of studies of bilingual aphasia, often focusing on describing symptoms, and on language localization (e.g., Fabro, 2001; Frenck-Mestre, Anton, Roth, Vaid, and Viallet, 2005; Mechelli, Crinion, et al., 2004). There have also been a number of chapters that summarize, debate, and review issues (e.g., Paradis,

2001; Roberts, 2001, 2007). Sadly, there have been very few studies of the reliability and validity of assessment tools, or of treatment outcomes for bilingual patients. This situation mirrors that in aphasiology as a whole, where studies of language localization and the nature of aphasia outnumber validation studies of tests and treatment studies (Roberts, Code, and McNeil, 2003). We are slowly adding to our knowledge on bilingual aphasia, but need a great deal more information about valid assessment, optimal treatment methods, and determining prognosis.

Assessment of Bilingual Aphasia

To assess a patient's post-stroke naming ability, clinicians and researchers may use subtests from one of the aphasia tests available in more than one language. These include the *Aachen Aphasia Test* (Graetz, de Bleser, and Willmes, 1992; Luzzati, Willmes, and de Bleser, 1992; Miller, de Bleser, and Willmes, 1997; Miller, Willmes, and de Bleser, 2000), the *Boston Diagnostic Aphasia Examination* (Goodglass and Kaplan, 1983; Goodglass, Kaplan, and Barresi, 2000; Laine, Goodglass, Niemi, Koivuselka-Sallinen, Tuomainen, and Martilla, 1993), the *Bilingual Aphasia Test* (BAT) (Paradis and Libben 1987; Juncos Rabadan, 1994; Juncos Rabadan, Elosua de Juan, Pereiro Rozas, and Torres Maroño, 1998) and the *Multilingual Aphasia Examination* (MAE) (Elias, Elias, D'Agostino, Silbershatz, and Wolf, 1997; Benton, Hamsher, and Sivan, 1994; Rey and Benton, 1991, 1999; Rey, Feldman, Hernandez, Levin, et al., 2001; Rey, Feldman, Rivas-Vazquez, Levin, and Benton, 1999). The psychometric properties of these tests in their various languages (their initial validity, test-retest reliability, available norms etc) vary widely, from one test to another and for different language versions of the same test. For example, there are norms for the English and Spanish MAE, but not for the French or German versions, nor for most versions of the BAT.

The problem of valid assessment in aphasia is particularly acute for bilingual aphasia, but extends to some of the English-language aphasia tests as well. For example, a recent U.S. government task force that reviewed only the BDAE, from among the tests listed above, found that "The *Boston Diagnostic Aphasia Examination*, 2nd Edition (BDAE-2) met neither the reliability nor validity criterion." (Agency for Health Care Research and Quality, 2002). They further identified the need for development of better tests for communication disorders, stating: "With the increasing cultural, linguistic, and racial diversity of the U.S. population, the applicability of assessment instruments to individuals who are members of different subpopulations is of crucial importance to clinical diagnosis and the process of disability determination. Despite the existence of a large number of speech and language assessment instruments, we still lack appropriate instruments for reliably and validly assessing speech and language in many subgroups defined in terms of language, dialect, or cultural differences. Thus, future research funding and priorities should be directed at addressing these serious deficiencies." (http://www.ahrq.gov/clinic/epcsums/spdissum.htm).

To measure change over time in a given patient, or in neurologically intact adults, any of the tests listed above could be used (although the sensitivity of some of them to detect change/differences has not been demonstrated). But to compare the post-stroke ability levels and the severity of the aphasia in each language of bilingual patients (i.e. how severe is the aphasia in Russian vs. in English?), it is vital to know to what extent the versions of a given test in each language are similar in their level of difficulty (Roberts, 1998a, 1998b, 2001, 2007). As we learn more about lexical, syntactic, and phonological processing, devising tests that are equivalent across languages becomes increasingly difficult. However, some basic criteria can be met, such as selecting stimuli for single word processing tasks that are equivalent in difficulty across languages. All of the aphasia tests published in different languages must be submitted to this time-consuming, yet vital process.

To assess naming ability, the *Boston Naming Test* (Kaplan, Goodglass, and Weintraub, 1983, 2001) has been studied in quite a range of languages including, for example, French (Roberts and Doucet, 2001; Roberts, Garcia, Desrochers, and Hernandez, 2002; Thuillard-Colombo and Assal, 1992), Spanish (Allegri, Mangone, Vallavicencio, Rymberg, Taragano, and Baumann, 1997; Kohnert, Hernandez, and Bates, 1998; Ponton, Satz, Herrera, et al., 1996; Ponton, Satz, Herrera, Young, Ortiz, D'Elia, et al., 1992), "Chinese" (Cheung, Cheung, and Chan, 2004), Dutch (Marien, Mampaey, Vervaet, Saerens, and DeDeyn, 1998), Finnish (Laine, Goodglass, Niemi, Koivuselka-Sallinen, Tuomainen, and Martilla, 1993), Greek (Tsolaki, Tsantali, Lekka, Kiosseoglou, and Kazis, 2003), Korean (Kim and Na, 1999), Norwegian (Hestad, Dybing, Haugen, and Klove, 1998), and Swedish (Tallberg, 2005). In most cases problems have been found with the level of name agreement: participants provided two or more different names for a picture included in the original BNT because the authors felt there was only one acceptable name in American English. Also, in the BNT studies that provide the item difficulty for all 60 items, the difficulty levels of some pictures for speakers of other languages do not follow the supposed order of difficulty for English (although the English pictures are not in order of difficulty for many unilingual English speakers (Roberts, Garcia, Desrochers, and Hernandez, 2002; Tombaugh and Hubley, 1997). In some cases, authors have changed so many of the original stimuli (for psychometric and cultural reasons) that the test is quite different in content from the original, English-language version of the BNT (Kim and Na, 1999).

Although there is no new test designed to assess bilingual aphasia, or bilingual naming impairments, there are now a number of sets of nouns (including but not limited to the Snodgrass and Vanderwart pictures) that have been tested in a range of languages for key features such as age of acquisition, length, frequency, imageability, and name agreement in French (e.g., Chalard, Bonin, Meot, Boyer, and Fayol, 1997; New, Pallier, Brysbaert, and Ferrand, 2004), in Italian (e.g., Barca, Burani, and Arduino, 2002), Icelandic (Pind, Joergen, Jonsdottir, Gossurardottir, and Jonsson, 2000) and in Spanish (e.g., Davis and Perea, 2005; Perez and Navalon, 2005).

There are two data bases of stimuli designed for use in a range of languages. Kremin, Akhutina, Basso, Davidoff, De Wilde, Kitzing, et al. (2003) have developed a set of 269 pictures, with normative data for 90 to 130 participants for each language, who were native speakers of Dutch, English, German, French, Italian, Russian, Spanish, and Swedish. Other work is underway expanding the list of languages and the types of French and Spanish (European vs. North American dialects). Szekely, Jacobsen, D'Amico, Devescovi, Andonova, Herron, et al., (2004; see also Szekely, D'Amico, Devescovi, Federmeier, Herron, Iyer, et al., 2005) have published results from the International Picture Naming Project (pictures and data are available at: http://crl.ucsd.edu/~aszekely/ipnp/) which provides data on 520 object names and 275 verbs in American English, German, Mexican Spanish, Italian, Bulgarian, Hungarian and a Taiwanese dialect of Mandarin. These data bases will facilitate future work on naming abilities in bilingual speakers, and the design of optimally valid and reliable assessments of bilingual aphasic adults.

The difficulties of assessing naming in bilingual speakers are not solved by comparing the performance of bilingual adults to that of unilingual speakers of each language or to groups of people who are described as "native speakers", since native speakers of one language often grow up to be bilingual or multilingual. There will always be differences from one bilingual speaker to the next, differences related to their own proficiency and acquisition history for each language. But, at least, if the same stimuli can be used across studies, stimuli with known psychometric properties, some of the potential causes of variance across studies can be reduced.

Alternate Assessment Methods for Expressive Language in Bilinguals

Given the problems of name agreement, and the impossibility of predicting the level of difficulty of any given picture for any given bilingual speaker, it may be helpful to consider more divergent types of tasks, especially generative naming. Advantages of verbal fluency tasks (also called generative naming) include the fact that no materials are required for the task and it can easily be administered in various language combinations (Roberts and Le Dorze, 1997). It has been repeatedly demonstrated that generative naming tasks are very sensitive to the effects of brain damage (see Spreen and Strauss, 1998) in aphasia, dementia and following right brain damage. There are studies of this task in quite a number of different countries and languages (e.g., Cardebat, Doyon, Puel, Goulet, and Joanette, 1990; Güven and Cangökçe, 2006; Roselli, Ardila, Salvatierra, Marquez, Matos, and Weekes, 2002; Snodgrass and Tsivkin, 1995; Tombaugh, Kozak, and Rees, 1999). These (and other similar) studies provide a frame of reference for interpreting the results, although when using verbal fluency to estimate a bilingual speaker's level of vocabulary knowledge, the key point is the difference in the number of words produced in each language, and not necessarily a comparison with normative samples of speakers of each language. The number of examples produced for common natural language categories such as animals, fruits, vegetables, foods, or clothing can be examined in each language, selecting semantic categories that take into account the patient's domains of use of each language. When scores on two or more different categories are combined, test-retest variability is reduced, and sensitivity is increased (Monsch, Bondi, Butters, Salmon, Katzman, and Thal, 1992; Roberts and Le Dorze, 1997).

Furthermore, in the domain of bilingual aphasia, Roberts and Le Dorze (1998) found similar performance across the two languages of French-English bilingual adults with aphasia and their controls, a finding partially replicated by Roselli (Roselli, Ardila, Salvatierra, Marquez, Matos, and Weekes, 2002).

Another divergent approach to estimating relative abilities in each language is to examine discourse production in patients with bilingual aphasia. Comparison of discourse samples in the two languages can provide qualitative information on word finding, code switching, and the types of word retrieval disturbances. The scoring system developed by Nicholas and Brookshire (1993) could be adapted for use with bilingual speakers. Muñoz and Marquardt (2004) examined several variables including the semantic accuracy of the utterance, the number of verbal disruptions (such as repetitions, omissions, fillers), and word retrieval errors (such as semantic errors, phonemic errors, descriptions). Munoz and Marquardt observed that two of their three bilingual aphasic patients demonstrated greater semantic accuracy and fewer paraphasias in English than in Spanish, whereas a third patient showed functional communication (very few errors) in the bilingual context.

Bilingual Aphasia Treatment Studies

Very few studies have addressed the issue of rehabilitation of language deficits in bilingual aphasia. Watamori and Sasanuma reported the effect of therapy on two patients with bilingual aphasia (Watamori and Sasanuma, 1976, 1978). One patient was a 69 year old, Japanese-English speaker, described as equally proficient but preferring to read and write in English. He suffered two CVAs and began speech therapy 2 months after the second one. He received therapy first in Japanese, from approximately 3 months post-onset (MPO) to 18 MPO, then therapy in both languages for a year. A second patient, 52 years old, probably spoke Japanese before he spoke English, although the authors note that the available information on his language history is incomplete. Starting at 3 MPO, he received six months of therapy in English.

Results revealed that the amount of recovery was greater in the trained language than the untrained language, although both patients improved to some degree in the untrained language. Specifically, Patient 1, who was assessed at 2, 14, 26 and 49 months after his stroke, demonstrated overall improvements in auditory comprehension, reading, and writing in both languages although oral production improved very little. Patient 2, who was assessed at 3, 7 and 9 months post onset, showed marginal improvements in auditory comprehension and reading but even less improvement in oral production and writing. Also, for both patients, differences in performance between the two languages in the four modalities (comprehension, reading, naming and writing) increased over time.

In both studies, it is impossible to separate the effects of the therapy early in the study from the spontaneous recovery, given how recent the strokes were. Information about language use and proficiency across modalities is incomplete, making it hard to interpret the reported scores in each language spoken by the two patients.

In another study, Sasanuma and Park (1995) examined one Korean-Japanese speaking individual (29 years old, L1-Korean, L2-Japanese, equally proficient, 2.5 months post onset) who received 36 sessions of treatment in Korean. The authors found equal levels of recovery in auditory and reading tasks in the treated and untreated language but greater improvements in Korean (the treated language) than Japanese on the oral production and writing tasks. However, it is not always the treated language that shows the greatest improvement (Roberts, 1992; Roberts, de la Riva, and Rhéaume, 1997).

Junque, Vendrell, Vendrell-Brucet, and Tobeña (1989) examined 30 Catalan-Spanish speaking individuals with aphasia. As Catalan was the more proficient language for all participants, treatment was provided in Catalan only. In all cases, improvement was greater in Catalan than in Spanish. While this study examined a fairly large number of bilingual patients, the nature of the language impairment was heterogeneous across the patients and the nature of therapy provided to the patients is relatively unclear.

Collectively, these studies provide evidence that the language of treatment influences recovery, but is not always the most important influence. Many more studies, including replications of published studies, will be needed to reveal how the many complex facets of bilingualism and aphasia interact to determine each patient's level of recovery in each language. These factors include the age of acquisition (AoA) and levels of proficiency in each modality in each language, the linguistic distance separating the patient's languages (e.g., English-Mandarin vs. Spanish-Italian), literacy levels in each language, aphasia types, the lesion size and site, the timing and intensity of therapy, and the methods used.

There are many important questions about whether treatment for bilingual aphasia generalizes across languages, to what extent, and why. Results of the few studies that have systematically examined naming treatment in individuals with bilingual aphasia show a range of patterns of crosslinguistic generalization. Hinckley (2003) provided treatment for naming deficits to a Spanish-English bilingual individual with aphasia (71 years, L1-Spanish, L2-English, 6 MPO). Using a cueing hierarchy treatment in English or Spanish did not yield crosslinguistic generalization as measured by the naming subtest of the *Bilingual Aphasia Test* (*BAT*) (Paradis and Libben, 1987). With no pre-stroke level of proficiency estimates, and the lack of studies to test the equivalency of the PALPA and the BAT in the two languages of this study (Spanish and English), the pretherapy and change scores are difficult to interpret.

In another study, Galvez and Hinckley (2003) used a cueing hierarchy with a balanced Spanish-English bilingual with transcortical motor aphasia (L1-Spanish, L2-English, late bilingual, 4 MPO). Language of treatment was alternated weekly. Overall improvement on the *BAT* was greater in Spanish than English, but naming scores on the *BAT* improved equally in the two languages.

Kohnert (2004) examined the effects of cognitive-based treatment and a lexical-based treatment on generalization in one bilingual patient with severe nonfluent aphasia (62 years old, L1-Spanish, L2-English, late bilingual, 4 MPO). Both treatments were effective in improving cognitive and language skills, measured in English and Spanish. The lexical-based therapy followed the cognitive therapy, in Spanish and then in English. Crosslinguistic (or between-language) generalization was reported for cognates (e.g., elephant/*elefante*) after the lexical therapy, but not for noncognates. Since the patient received treatment for both languages without a true control condition, it is not clear to what extent these improvements are caused by some aspect of one or both therapies or by the patient having named the pictures repetitively (Kohnert, 2004).

These bilingual aphasia treatment studies demonstrate the importance of adequately describing each patient (see also Roberts, Code, and McNeil, 2003), their language levels pre-stroke, and of using tests and stimuli that have known properties (to the extent possible). When it has not been possible to use tests or stimuli with demonstrated cross-language equivalence, authors and readers must be very cautious in the conclusions they draw from their results. As more bilingual aphasic adults are studied, patterns in treatment outcomes may emerge, but we will be able to see the patterns only if each patient is described in more detail than is currently common practice.

In a recent study, crosslinguistic generalization patterns were systematically examined in three English-Spanish bilingual individuals with aphasia (Edmonds and Kiran, 2006). Results revealed crosslinguistic generalization in all participants. However, the patterns of generalization differed across participants. The first patient (P1) in this open-ended series was pre-morbidly equally proficient in English and Spanish. Training in Spanish resulted in improved ability to name trained items (e.g., *manzana*) and within language generalization to semantically related items (e,g., *naranja*) (*manzana* means "apple" and *naranja* means "orange"). Additionally, crosslinguistic generalization was observed on untrained semantically related items (e.g., *orange*) with marginal improvement on the untrained English translation equivalents of trained Spanish items (e.g., *apple*). As predicted, no appreciable gains were observed in the Spanish and English control words (untreated and semantically unrelated to the treatment stimuli), indicating that observed improvements were due to treatment.

Patients 2 and 3 (P2 and P3) were both pre-morbidly more proficient in English than in Spanish. Whereas P2 first received treatment in English followed by Spanish, P3 received treatment in Spanish only. With English treatment, P2 showed improvements on trained items (e.g., *apple*), within-language generalization to semantically related items (e.g., *orange*) within the more proficient language but no crosslinguistic generalization. However, when treatment was shifted to Spanish (the less proficient language), improvement of trained items was observed (e,g., *naranja*), but within-language generalization to semantically related untrained items (e.g., *manzana*) was not observed. Importantly, with Spanish treatment, crosslinguistic generalization was observed for English translation equivalents and corresponding semantically related items. These results were replicated in P3, who was also more proficient in English. The main finding of this study was that crosslinguistic generalization was observed in all participants. P1, who was pre-morbidly equally proficient across languages, was trained in Spanish and showed generalization to English. P2 and P3 were pre-morbidly more proficient in English but, when trained in Spanish, showed generalization to English.

In a follow-up study by Kiran and Roberts, three additional aphasic adults, two English-Spanish speakers and one French-English speaker have been studied to date. As the *n* gradually increases, we hope to be able to make progressively more informed interpretations of why generalization within and/or between languages occurs for some patients and not for others.

Methodological Issues

To conduct a study of the effects of therapy on any component of language in bilingual aphasic adults, a number of methodological challenges must be met. Given the current state of knowledge and the variation across different bilingual speakers, it is impossible to meet all of these challenges with a high level of rigor, but researchers need to be aware of the challenges, and do everything possible to move closer to meeting them as our knowledge base expands. Readers of research need to be aware of these challenges as they evaluate the quality of published studies and try to apply published results to their own clinical work. The strategies proposed below for responding to these challenges are not "solutions", but ways to reduce the impact of factors that weaken the validity of tests and therapy studies and thus make interpretation of the results problematic.

Among the challenges in conducting studies of bilingual aphasia are the following:

1. The complexity of aphasia and our incomplete understanding of it: In reading and interpreting studies of bilingual aphasia treatment, it is vital to remember that there is great variability inherent in aphasia. The treatment studies on unilingual speakers show that a given therapy will help some patients but not others, even when these patients seem to be "the same" i.e. have a similar aphasia type and/or severity and/or time post-onset, and/or lesion location. In other studies, all patients will improve but the extent of improvement will be much greater in some patients than in others. Some unilingual patients generalize treatment gains across modalities, while others do not. Some unilingual patients generalize treatment gains to untreated words or structures, while others do not. In some cases, readers can find these disparate outcomes within a single study (e.g., Laganaro, Di Pietro, and Schnider, 2006; Nettleton and Lesser, 1991); in other cases, it is by comparing one study to another that one sees the range of outcomes. Possible explanations for the varied response to treatment include the severity of the aphasia, the exact nature of the impairment, the functional importance of spared vs. damaged regions or networks within each patient's brain and the combined effects of pre-stroke proficiency in each language and the deficits (parallel or otherwise) caused by the stroke. In studies of bilingual aphasia, if one patient or group or type of word improves and the others do not, there is a tendency to interpret results in terms of the bilingualism: early vs. late acquisition; level of proficiency, etc. The features of each patient's bilingualism are important, but they are not the only – and sometimes probably not even the most important – explanatory variables.

One way to help isolate what is due to bilingualism and what is due to the aphasia would be to include unilingual and bilingual patients in the same study. By comparing the symptoms or the treatment outcomes of one or more bilingual patients to the symptoms or outcomes of one or more unilingual patients, the patterns of deficits, improvement, and generalization (or lack thereof) can be better understood and, over a series of studies, the impact of bilingualism can be isolated. A second strategy is to use a larger number of patients in each study. The larger the number of participants, the more chance there is to see patterns and to accurately interpret results.

A third remedy is for all researchers in aphasia to provide more information about their patients (see Roberts, Code, and McNeil, 2003; Roberts, Code, Hillis, and McNeil, forthcoming). Obtaining careful pre-morbid language proficiency information is as important as the pre-treatment language assessment for these patients. In bilingual aphasia, the information provided about each patient's bilingual history and proficiency still varies widely from one article to the next and is usually incomplete. This makes it impossible to compare patients across studies, since we do not know in what ways they may be similar. The BAT contains a very thorough, detailed language history questionnaire (Paradis and Libben, 1987).

Roberts and Shenker have published a somewhat shorter history form that can be used with any research participant or clinical patient (Roberts and Shenker, 2007). In Table 2, we list the information that all authors should provide about the language background of their participants. If journal reviewers and editors adopted this list (or a similar one) as part of the requirements for all papers on bilingual adults, it would contribute significantly to progress in studies of bilingualism and of bilingual aphasia. We welcome discussion and suggestions on this issue.

Table 1. Challenges and suggested strategies to meet them.

Challenge	Mitigating strategy or response
1. the complexity of aphasia; no two patients the same	Study bilingual and unilingual patients in the same study to partially isolate effects of bilingualism vs. effects of aphasia; more complete description of each participant's language status; larger n in each study; replicate studies.
2. pre-stroke proficiency levels affect post-stroke performance, yet are unknowable	Estimate pre-stroke levels through combination of language history, domains of use, and self-ratings and/or family ratings of proficiency in each modality.
3. variability and unknowns in each adult's pre-stroke vocabulary	More complete descriptions of each person's proficiency; select stimuli with known psychometric properties, to the extent possible; larger n in each study; replicate studies; have a group of adults with similar language histories perform the experimental or therapy tasks to provide a reference range for interpreting patients' performance.
4. practice effects may affect scores on some tasks when testing two or more languages	Studies to measure this on various tests and tasks; retest in the same language to be able to compare within-language TRT changes to between-language differences. See Roberts 1998a
5. fatigue	Monitor length of sessions; look for signs of fatigue; provide breaks; ask patient !
6. cognates may make some tasks easier for pairs of languages where they exist	Control stimuli to eliminate cognate pairs or include sets of cognate words and non-cognate words, matched for length, frequency etc and compare results on the two types of words; verify cognateness by asking speakers of the pairs of languages to be used in the study.

Finally, replications of already-published studies are needed using the same pairs of languages and different ones. Patterns of deficits or therapy effects that occur in Dutch-

English bilinguals might or might not be replicated in Punjabi-Arabic or Russian-English speakers.

As we strive to better understand cross-language generalization in aphasia treatment, it is helpful to consider the literature on cross-language generalization of gains in treatment in other disorders, where similar questions are being studied (e.g., Holm and Dodd, 2001; Jordaan, Shaw-Ridley, Serfontein, Orelowitz, and Monaghan, 2001; McNutt, 1994). Studies of response to treatment for other disorders in bilingual children and adults may have useful findings that can help in understanding bilingual aphasia treatment.

2. Pre-stroke levels of proficiency: Neuroimaging studies show that cortical areas activated during lexical tasks largely overlap in a bilingual brain. But it remains unknown to what extent this gross anatomical overlap implies that the two languages are processed by the same micro level networks (Crinion et al., 2006; Roberts, 2001; Steinmetz and Seitz, 1991). AoA seems to influence localization with less overlap occurring for the two languages if one of them is acquired much later than the other (e.g., Dehaene et al., 1997; Kim et al., 1997). However, level of proficiency may be at least as important (Abutalebi, Cappa, and Perani, 2001), and cumulative exposure is also a factor (Perani, et al., 2003). We must remain cautious in interpreting "localization studies" using fMRI, given the constraints imposed on participants during the testing, the few patients and pairs of languages tested, the limited tasks performed, and the range of possible interpretations of results such as "more activation" or "less activation" in specific regions (see Van Lancker Sidtis, 2006 for a skeptical review of these and other issues about fMRI).

Table 2. Essential information for describing the language background of participants in studies of bilingual aphasia.

1. List of languages the patient/participant (P) could understand;
2. Age of first regular exposure to each language identified in Question 1: classes in school; radio or TV; moved to new country or city; new friends or activities that exposed P to a new language;
3. Percent of use of each language in adulthood for at least the following domains: home life, work, socializing, reading, television/radio. A rough idea of the main language(s) used in childhood is also helpful, if P or the family can provide this. However, the farther back in time you probe, the less accurate the information MAY be, for some patients.
4. How each language was learned: relative roles of informal acquisition and classroom study.
5. Changes in overall patterns of use over P's lifetime i.e. was there a time when P used only one language? Or used a language that he has not had to use for many years?
6. Estimates of proficiency: obtained from family members and/or from P, if able.

A 7-point scale works well and is often used in studies of non-aphasic bilinguals. It works best with an added 0 (making an 8-point scale), because it seems to confuse people to rate something as a 1, yet mean "zero ability or knowledge". Several versions of this scale and various forms of instructions have been used by Roberts and by other authors. The current version developed at the University of Ottawa is provided in Appendix A.

To estimate pre-stroke levels of proficiency, some authors have used naming time (e.g., Langdon, Wiig, and Nielson, 2005); some have used the lexical decision task as a measure of language proficiency (Lemhöfer, Dijkstra, and Michel, 2004). But the most common way of providing information about likely pre-stroke levels of proficiency has been to describe the participant's language history. The information required includes: 1) language acquisition: age began learning each L, methods; 2) domains of use – a patient's family can often provide this information; 3) estimated proficiency by the patient, if the aphasia is mild enough to allow this, and/or by one or more bilingual family members. The accuracy of these self-ratings and of family ratings is unknown, but they have proved to yield "higher level" and "lower level" groups of participants in a number of studies where they have been used (Roberts and Le Dorze, 1997; Roberts and Bois, 1999). Self-ratings may be more accurate in some situations, for some levels of ability than for others (Delgado, Guerrero, Goggin, and Ellis, 1999; Dunning and Kruger, 1999; Langdon, Wiig, and Nielson, 2005).

For the rating task, a 7 point scale, with the end-points defined can be used (see Table 2 for more details on the rating). Alternatively, patients/families can rate each modality as "a little better" or "a lot better" (as in Roberts and Le Dorze, 1997, 1998). In these studies, patients and families were asked: *No one ever has exactly the same level in their two languages, but would you say that he spoke/understood/read/wrote _____ and _____ at roughly the same level or was one language better than the other?* If they say one was better, ask: *was it a LOT better, or just a LITTLE better?* One suggested addition to these ratings is to ask: Why do you say it was better, in what way was it better? This can help them think about vocabulary, grammar, accent, rate of speech, etc. and help the interviewer understand the framework that the family member or patient is using for their ratings.

3. Assessing the extent of the naming deficit: In bilingual adults post-stroke, it is impossible to know what words their pre-morbid lexicon in each language contained. It is now clear that both age of acquisition (AoA) and, probably to a lesser extent, frequency of occurrence in each language affect naming speed, lexical decision speed and accuracy, and performance on other lexical processing tasks, although the relationship between these (and other) variables is still being probed (e.g., Ghyselinck, Lewis, and Brysbaert, 2004; Johnston, and Barry, 2006 for recent reviews; Lehtonen and Laine, 2003; Voyer, 2003). In individual bilingual speakers, it is very difficult (perhaps impossible?) to know the AoA for items on naming tests or in sets of stimuli. The studies on the *Boston Naming Test* cited above demonstrate how the performance of speakers across languages and across cultures varies. An unknown number of the speakers in these studies were bilingual or multilingual. This makes interpreting the results of these studies even more problematic.

Given the complementarity principle - the use of languages in various domains and for different communication tasks based on need and exposure (Grosjean, 1998) – we can expect most speakers to have non-equivalent vocabularies in their two languages. Therefore, it is impossible to know when a particular item is not named whether this is due to the aphasia or to pre-morbid vocabulary "holes". If some words were known in both languages pre-stroke, but in the weaker language the word was acquired as an adult and/or rarely used, does this make it more vulnerable to anomia?

There is no easy solution to the problems created by the non-equivalency of the items in the test in terms of their frequency of occurrence and typical AoA for unilingual speakers and the unknown frequency of occurrence, and age-of-acquisition for each bilingual speaker. One approach is to test the stimuli to be used with patients on a group of non-aphasic bilingual speakers from the same community. For a confrontation naming task, Croft, Marshall, and Pring (2006) selected stimuli presented to 6 Bengali-English bilingual aphasic adults based on the naming latencies and name agreement obtained from a group of 20 Bengali-English speaking, non-aphasic adults. To the extent that stimuli are prepared based on known AoA, name agreement, frequency of occurrence and the other factors identified in studies of lexical access in various languages, some of the "noise" in data from bilingual studies can be reduced.

4. Practice effects and other threats to test-retest reliability: When the two languages are tested on the same day, often in the same clinical session, is there is a practice effect (see Roberts, 1998a, 2001)? Does testing on different days make a practice effect more or less likely? On the 30-item Graded Naming Test (McKenna and Warrington, 1983), some non-aphasic adults improved their score by 1 to 2 items, resulting in a change in the mean group score of 1 point (Roberts, 2003). Brain damage probably makes a practice effect less likely. Cooper and colleagues (2001) found no practice effect for patients with dementia on a category verbal fluency task. However, in aphasic adults, Roberts and Le Dorze (1994) found slight improvements in verbal fluency on retesting. Even in those patients with chronic aphasia (at least one year post-onset), the individual participants' change scores (test 2 − test 1) ranged from -6 to + 9. Note that this problem is not unique to bilingual aphasia, nor even to communication disorders. Some quite widely-used tests fail to meet acceptable levels of test-retest reliability (e.g., Philp, Lowles, Armstrong, and Whitehead, 2002). Nonetheless, it is a problem that needs to be better understood if we are to interpret differences in scores across languages, and also changes in scores from pre- to post-therapy.

5. Fatigue: Because of the effects of the stroke, fatigue during aphasia testing is often a problem. Fatigue can lead to lower scores when a patient is tested on a "bad day" or after completing other tests. Given that bilingual aphasic patients must be tested in each language, the testing is, unavoidably, longer and therefore more tiring. To mitigate this, frequent breaks and shorter blocks of testing may help.

6. Cognates: Cognates are pairs of words with the same meaning in two (or more) languages and similar pronunciation and/or spelling. There is still no consensus on how close in spelling or pronunciation a pair of words must be to count as cognates. But there is now a body of studies using different language pairs, showing consistent differences between the processing time, priming effects and task accuracy for cognates compared to non-cognates on a range of tasks (e.g., Costa, Caramazza, and Sebastian-Galles, 2000; Costa, Santesteban, and Caño, 2005; de Groot, 1993; Gollan, Forster, and Frost, 1997). If tests such as the BNT are simply translated, and administered in the patients' two languages, there is no control over the number of cognates that will arise for any given pair of languages. For French-English and Spanish-English speakers, the BNT produces approximately 20 cognates out of the 60 pictures (the exact number would depend on how "cognate" was defined and which synonyms/dialectal variants are accepted). But for other pairs of languages, there might be no cognate pairs. So, the difficulty of this test is reduced for speakers of languages with higher numbers of cognate stimuli. For language pairs where there happen to be few or no cognate stimuli, the test may be more difficult.

Moreover, cognates may have a facilitative effect on word retrieval in patients with bilingual aphasia, presumably due to the overlapping phonology across the two languages. For instance, using a picture naming task, Roberts and Deslauriers (1999) found that cognate pictures were more often correctly named in both languages than non-cognates in both normal English-French bilinguals and in 10 patients with bilingual aphasia. Likewise, Lalor and Kirsner (2001) found that a 63-year-old Italian-English bilingual individual with aphasia performed better on cognates in both languages. Cognates may also facilitate cross-language generalization in language treatment (Kohnert, 2004).

We recommend excluding cognate words from naming tests and treatment stimuli or reporting separately on the results for cognates and non-cognates.

Summary and Conclusion

As the field of bilingual aphasia grows, our understanding of the nature of bilingual aphasia is expanding. For both clinical and research purposes, there is an urgent need to develop psychometrically stronger assessment tools. Given the complex nature of bilingualism and of aphasia, and the variability across bilingual speakers, it is difficult to know why a given patient may fail a particular task, such as naming a particular picture. However, by using experimental tasks and tests that take into account what is now known about the lexicon and lexical processing, we can significantly improve the validity of studies of bilingual naming and bilingual aphasia therapy. We urge researchers to provide much more detailed and more uniform descriptions of each participant's language history and to try to control for more potentially confounding factors in the choice of stimuli, assessment tools, and therapy designs.

We urge readers to be critical in reading published studies that fail to provide key information about the participants, and call on authors to be more circumspect in drawing conclusions from their own data, given the variability inherent in both aphasia and bilingualism and the difficulty in controlling the many factors that can influence test results and treatment outcomes in bilingual aphasia.

References

Abutalebi, J. Cappa, S. F. & Perani, D. (2001). The bilingual brain as revealed by functional neuroimaging. *Bilingualism: Language and Cognition, 4*, 179-190.

Agency for Healthcare Research and Quality. (2002). *Criteria for Determining Disability in Speech-Language Disorders*. Summary, Evidence Report/Technology Assessment:

Number 52. AHRQ Publication No. 02-E009, January 2002., Rockville, MD. http://www.ahrq.gov/clinic/epcsums/spdissum.htm

Allegri, R. F., Mangone, C. A., Villavicencio, A. F., Rymberg, S., Taragano, F. E. & Baumann, D. (1997). Spanish Boston Naming Test norms. *The Clinical Neuropsychologist, 11*, 416-420.

Barca, L., Burani, C. & Arduino, L. S. (2002). Word naming times and psycholinguistic norms for Italian nouns. *Behavior Research Methods, Instruments, and Computers, 34(3),* 424-434.

Benton, A. L., Hamsher, K. S. & Sivan, A. B. (1994). *Multilingual Aphasia Examination, 3rd Edition (MAE).* Iowa City: AJA Associates.

Butler, Y. G. & Hakuta, K. (2006). Bilingualism and second language acquisition. In: K. Bhatia, & W. C. Ritchie (Eds.), *The handbook of bilingualism* (114-144). Malden, MA: Blackwell Publishing.

Cardebat, D., Doyon, B., Puel, M., Goulet, P. & Joanette, Y. (1990). Evocation lexicale formelle et sémantique chez des sujets normaux : performances et dynamique de production en fonction du sexe, de l'âge, et du niveau d'étude. *Acta Neurologica Belgica, 90,* 207-217.

Chalard, M., Bonin, P., Meot, A, Boyer, B. & Fayol, M. (1997). Objective age-of-acquisition (AoA) norms for a set of 230 object names in French: Relationships with psycholinguistic variables, the English data from Morrison et al. (1997), and naming latencies. *European Journal of Cognitive Psychology, 15,* 209-245.

Cheung, R. W., Cheung, M. C. & Chan, A. S. (2004). Confrontation naming in Chinese patients with left, right or bilateral brain damage. *Journal of the International Neuropsychological Society, 10,* 46-53.

Christophersen, P. (1999). Two more contributions to the nativeness debate. *RASK Supplement, 9,* 117-122.

Cooper, D. B., Epker, M., Lacritz, L.,Weiner, M., Rosenberg, R. N., Honig, L. & Cullum, C. M. (2001). Effects of practice on category fluency in Alzheimer's disease. *Clinical Neuropsychologist, 15,* 125-128.

Costa, A., Caramazza, A. & Sebastian-Galles, N. (2000). The cognate facilitation effect: implications for models of lexical access. *Journal of Experimental Psychology: Learning, Memory and Cognition, 26(5),* 1283-1296.

Costa, A., Santesteban, M. & Caño, A. (2005). On the facilitatory effects of cognate words in bilingual speech production. *Brain and Language, 94,* 94-103.

Crinion, J., Turner, R., Grogan, A., Hanakawa, T., Noppeney, U., Devlin, J. T., Aso, T., Urayama, S., Fukuyama, H., Stockton, K., Usui, K., Green, D. W. & Price, C. J. (2006). Language control in the bilingual brain. *Science, 312(5779),* 1537-1540.

Croft, Marshall, J. & Pring, T. (2006). Assessing noun naming impairments in bilingual aphasia. *Brain and Language, 99,* 21-22.

Davis, C. J. & Perea, M. (2005). Per BuscaPalabras: A program for deriving orthographic and phonological neighborhood statistics and other psycholinguistic indices in Spanish. *Behavior Research Methods, 37,* 665-671.

De Bot, K. (2004). The multilingual lexicon: modelling selection and control. *International Journal of Multilingualism, 1,* 17-32.

De Groot, A. M. B. (1993). Word-type effects in bilingual processing tasks : Support for a mixed representational system. In R. Schreuder and B. Weltens (Eds.), *The bilingual lexicon* (27-51). Amsterdam: Elsevier.

Dehaene, S., Dupoux, E., Mehler, J., Cohen, L., Paulesu, E., Perani, D., Van de Moortele, P. F., Lehericy, S. & Le Bihan, D. (1997). Anatomical variability in the cortical representation of first and second language. *NeuroReport, 8*, 3809-3815.

Delgado, P., Guerrero, G., Goggin, J. P. & Ellis, B. B. (1999). Self-assessment of linguistic skills by bilingual Hispanics. *Hispanic Journal of Behavioral Sciences, 21(1)*, 31-46.

Dijkstra, T., del Prado M., Fermin M., Schulpen, B., Schreuder, R. & Baayen, R. H. (2005). A roommate in cream: Morphological family size effects on interlingual homograph recognition. *Language and Cognitive Processes, 20*, 7-41.

Dunning, D. & Kruger, J. (1999). Unskilled and unaware of it: how difficulties in recognizing one's own incompetence lead to inflated self-assessments. *Journal of Personality and Social Psychology, 77*, 1121-1134.

Edmonds, L. A. & Kiran, S. (2006). Effect of semantic based treatment on cross linguistic generalization in bilingual aphasia. *Journal of Speech, Language, and Hearing Research, 49*, 729-748.

Edwards, J. (2006). Foundations of bilingualism. In: T. K. Bhatia, & W. C. Ritchie (Eds.), *The handbook of bilingualism* (7-31). Malden, MA: Blackwell Publishing.

Elias, M. F., Elias, P. K., D'Agostino, R. B., Silbershatz, H. & Wolf, P. A. (1997). Role of age, education, and gender on cognitive performance in the Framingham Heart Study: Community-based norms. *Experimental Aging Research, 23*, 201-235.

Fabbro, F. (2001). The bilingual brain: Cerebral representation of languages. *Brain and Language, 79*, 211-222.

Frenck-Mestre, C., Anton, J. L., Roth, M., Vaid, J. & Viallet, F. (2005). Articulation in early and late bilinguals' two languages: evidence from functional magnetic resonance imaging. *Neuroreport, 16*, 761-765.

Galvez, A. & Hinckley, J. J. (2003). Transfer patterns of naming treatment in a case of bilingual aphasia. *Brain and Language, 87*, 173-174.

Ghyselinck, M., Lewis, M. B. & Brysbaert, M. (2004). Age of acquisition and the cumulative-frequency hypothesis: A review of the literature and a new multi-task investigation. *Acta Psychologica, 115*, 43-67.

Gollan, T. H., Forster, K. I. & Frost, R. (1997). Translation priming with different scripts: masked priming with cognates and non-cognates in Hebrew-English bilinguals. *Journal of Experimental Psychology: Learning, Memory, and Cognition, 23*, 1122-1139.

Goodglass, H. & Kaplan, E. (1983). *The Boston Diagnostic Aphasia Examination.* Philadelphia: Lea and Febiger.

Goodglass, H., Kaplan, E. and Barresi, B. (2000). *The Boston Diagnostic Aphasia Examination. 3rd edition.* Austin, TX: Pro-Ed.

Goral, M., Levy, E. S., Obler, L. K. & Cohen, E. (2006). Cross-language lexical connections in the mental lexicon: Evidence from a case of trilingual aphasia. *Brain and Language, 98*, 235-247.

Goral, M. & Obler, L. K. (in press) Two's company, three's a crowd? Recent advances in psycholinguistic and neurolinguistic study of multilingual speakers. In: A. Stavans, &

I. Kupferberg (Eds.), Studies in language and language education: *Essays in honor of Elite Olshtain*. Jerusalem: The Hebrew University Magnes Press.

Graetz, P., de Bleser, R. & Willmes, K. (1992). *Akense afasie test*. Lisse, The Netherlands: Swetz and Zeitlinger. (Aachen Aphasia Test)

Grosjean, F. (1989). Neurolinguists beware! The bilingual is not two monolinguals in one person. *Brain and Language, 36*, 3-15.

Grosjean, F. (1998). Studying bilinguals: methodological and conceptual issues. *Bilingualism: Language and Cognition, 1,* 131-149.

Güven, A. G. & Cangökçe, O. (2006). The role of education levels and gender on reading and phonemic (initial letter) fluency in healthy adults. Türk Psikologi Dergisi, *21(57)*, 121-123 (English summary) (and 109-120, full article).

Harris, R. J. (Ed.) (1992). *Cognitive processing in bilinguals*. New York: Elsevier.

Hestad, K., Dybing, E., Haugen, P. K. & Klove, H. (1998). Using the Boston Naming Test to assess anomic difficulties in patients with dementia. [Norwegian]. Original Title Sprakforstyrrelser hos demente pasienter undersokt med Boston Naming Test. Tidsskrift for Norsk Psykologforening, 35, 322-327. English abstract in PsychInfo.

Hinckley, J. J. (2003). Picture naming treatment in aphasia yields greater improvement in L1. *Brain and Language, 87*, 171-172.

Holm A. & Dodd B. (2001). Comparison of cross-language generalisation following speech therapy. *Folia Phoniatrica et Logopaedica, 53*, 166-172.

Hyltenstam, K. (1992). Non-native features of near-native speakers: on the ultimate attainment of childhood L2 learners. In: R. J. Harris (Ed.), *Cognitive processing in bilinguals* (351-368). New York: Elsevier.

Johnston, R. A. & Barry, C. (2006). Age of acquisition and lexical processing. *Visual Cognition, 13*, 789-845.

Jordaan, H., Shaw-Ridley, G, Serfontein, J., Orelowitz, K. & Monaghan, N. (2001). Cognitive and linguistic profiles of specific language impairment and semantic-pragmatic disorder in bilinguals. *Folia Phoniatrica et Logopaedica, 53*,153-165.

Juncos Rabadan, O. (1994). The assessment of bilingualism in normal aging with the Bilingual Aphasia Test. *Journal of Neurolinguistics, 8*, 67-73.

Juncos Rabadan, O. and Iglesias, (1994). Decline in the elderly's language: Evidence from cross-linguistic data. *Journal of Neurolinguistics, 8(3)*, 183-190.

Juncos Rabadan, O., Elosua de Juan, R., Pereiro Rozas, A. & Torres Marono, M. (1998). Lexical difficulties in the elderly: Basis for intervention.[Spanish].(Problemas de acceso lexico en la vejez. Bases para la intervencion. *Anales de Psicologia, 4*, 169-176.

Junque, C., Vendrell, P., Vendrell-Brucet, J. M. & Tobeña, A. (1989). Differential recovery in naming in bilingual aphasics. *Brain and Language, 36*, 16-22.

Kaplan, E., Goodglass, H. & Weintraub, S. (1983). *The Boston Naming Test*. Philadelphia: Lea and Febiger.

Kaplan, E., Goodglass, H. & Weinbraub. S. (2001). *The Boston Naming Test. 2nd edition*. Baltimore: Lippincott, Williams and Wilkins.

Kim, H. & Na, D. L. (1999). Normative data on the Korean version of the Boston Naming Test. *Journal of Clinical and Experimental Neuropsychology, 21*, 127-133.

Kim, K. H. S., Relkin, N. R., Lee, K. M. & Hirsch, J. (1997). Distinct cortical areas associated with native and second languages. *Nature, 388*, 171-174.

Kohnert, K. (2004). Cognitive and cognate-based treatments for bilingual aphasia: a case study. *Brain and Language, 91*, 294-302.

Kohnert, K. J., Hernandez, A. E. & Bates, E. (1998). Bilingual performance on the Boston Naming Test: Preliminary norms in Spanish and English. *Brain and Language, 65*, 422-440.

Kremin, H., Akhutina, T., Basso, A., Davidoff, J., De Wilde, M., Kitzing, P., et al. (2003). A cross-linguistic data bank for oral picture naming in Dutch, English, German, French, Italian, Russian, Spanish, and Swedish (PEDOI). *Brain and Cognition, 53*, 243-246.

Laganaro, M., Di Pietro, M. & Schnider, A. (2006). What does recovery from anomia tell us about the underlying impairment: the case of similar anomic patterns and different recovery. *Neuropsychologia, 44,* 534-545.

Laine, M., Goodglass, H., Niemi, J., Koivuselka-Sallinen, P., Tuomainen, J. & Martilla, R. (1993). Adaptation of the Boston Diagnostic Aphasia Examination and the Boston Naming Test into Finnish. *Scandinavian Journal of Logopedics and Phoniatrics, 18*, 83-92.

Lalor, E. & Kirsner, K. (2001). The role of cognates in bilingual aphasia: Implications for assessment and treatment. *Aphasiology, 15(10)*, 1047-1056.

Langdon, H. W., Wiig, E. H. & Nielson, N. P. (2005). Dual-dimension naming speed and language-dominance ratings by bilingual Hispanic adults. *Bilingual Research Journal, 29*, 319-336.

Lehtonen, M. & Laine, M. (2003). How word frequency affects morphological processing in monolinguals and bilinguals. *Bilingualism: Language and Cognition, 6*, 213-225.

Lemhöfer, K., Dijkstra, T. & Michel, M. C. (2004). Three languages, one ECHO: Cognate effects in trilingual word recognition. *Language and Cognitive Processes, 19*, 585-611.

Levey, S. (2004). Discrimination and production of English vowels by bilingual speakers of Spanish and English. *Perceptual and Motor Skills, 99,* 445-462.

Luzzati, C., Willmes, K. & de Bleser, R. (1992). *Aachener Aphasie Test: versione italiana.* Firenze: O.S. Organizzazioni Speciali. (The Aachen Aphasia Test.)

Marien, P., Mampaey, E., Vervaet, A., Saerens, J. & De Deyn, P. P. (1998). Normative data for the Boston Naming Test in native Dutch-speaking Belgian elderly. *Brain and Language, 65*, 447-467.

McKenna, P. & Warrington, E. K. (1983). *The Graded Naming Test.* Windsor, UK: NFER-Nelson.

McNutt, J. C. (1994). Generalization of /s/ from English to French as a result of phonological remediation. *Journal of Speech Language Pathology and Audiology, 18*, 109-113.

Mechelli, A., Crinion, J. T., Noppeney, U., O'Doherty, J., Ashburner, J., Frackowiak, R. S. & Price, C. J. (2004). Structural plasticity in the bilingual brain: Proficiency in a second language and age at acquisition affect grey-matter density. *Nature, 431(7010)*, 757.

Miller, N., de Bleser, R. & Willmes, K. (1997). The English language version of the Aachen Aphasia Test, In: W. Ziegler, & K. Deger (Eds.), *Clinical Phonetics and Linguistics* (257-265). London: Whurr.

Miller, N., Willmes, K. & De Bleser, R. (2000). The psychometric properties of the English language version of the Aachen Aphasia Test (EEAT). *Aphasiology, 14,* 683-722.

Monsch, A., Bondi, M., Butters, N., Salmon,D., Katzman, R. & Thal, L. (1992). Comparison of verbal fluency tasks in the detection of dementia of the Alzheimer type. *Archives of Neurology, 49,* 1253-1258.

Muñoz, M. L. & Marquardt, T. P. (2004). The influence of language context on lexical retrieval in the discourse of bilingual speakers with aphasia. *Journal of Multilingual Communication Disorders, 2,* 1-17.

Nettleton, J. & Lesser, R. (1991). Therapy for naming difficulties in aphasia: application of a cognitive neuropsychological model. *Journal of Neurolinguistics, 6,* 139-157.

New, B., Pallier, C., Brysbaert, M. & Ferrand, L. (2004). Lexique 2: A new French lexical database. *Behavior Research Methods, Instruments and Computers, 36(3),* 516-524.

Newman, R. S. & German, D.J. (2005). Life span effects of lexical factors on oral naming. *Language and Speech, 48,* 123-156.

Nicholas, N. E. & Brookshire, R. H. (1993). A system for quantifying the informativeness and efficiency of the connected speech of adults with aphasia. *Journal of Speech and Hearing Research, 36,* 338-350.

Paradis, M. (1995). Bilingual aphasia 100 years later: consensus and controversies. In: M. Paradis (Ed.), *Aspects of bilingual aphasia* (211-223). Tarrytown, NY: Elsevier.

Paradis, M. (2001). In: R. S. Berndt (Ed). *Handbook of neuropsychology,* 2nd ed.: Vol 3: *Language and aphasia.* (69-91). Amsterdam: Elsevier Science Publishers.

Paradis, M. & Libben, G. (1987). *The assessment of bilingual aphasia.* Hillsdale, NJ: Lawrence Erlbaum Associates.

Pavlenko, A. (2000). L2 influence on L1 in late bilingualism. *Issues in Applied Linguistics, 11,* 175-205.

Pavlenko, A. & Jarvis, S. (2002). Bidirectional transfer. *Applied Linguistics, 23,* 190-214. Perani, D., Abutalebi, J., Paulesu, E., Brambati, S., Scifo, P., Cappa, S. F. & Fazio, F. (2003). The role of age of acquisition and language usage in early, high-proficient bilinguals: an fMRI study during verbal fluency. *Human Brain Mapping, 19(3),* 170-182.

Perez, M. A. & Navalon, C. (2005). Objective-AoA norms for 175 names in Spanish: Relationships with other psycholinguistic variables, estimated AoA, and data from other languages. *European Journal of Cognitive Psychology, 17,* 179-206.

Philp, I., Lowles, R. V., Armstrong, G. K. & Whitehead, C. (2002). Repeatability of standardized tests of functional impairment and well-being in older people in a rehabilitation setting. *Disability and Rehabilitation, 24(5),* 243-249.

Pind, J., Jonsdottir, H., Gossurardottir, H. & Jonsson, F. (2000). Icelandic norms for the Snodgrass and Vanderwart (1980) pictures: Name and image agreement, familiarity, and age of acquistion. *Scandinavian Journal of Psychology, 41(1),* 41-48.

Ponton, M. O., Satz, P., Herrera, L., et al. (1996). Normative data stratified by age and education for the Neuropsychological Screening Battery for Hispanics (NeSBHIS): Initial report. *Journal of the International Neuropsychological Societ, 2,* 96-104.

Ponton, M. O., Satz, P., Herrera, L., Young, R., Ortiz, F., D'Elia, L. et al. (1992). Modified Spanish version of the Boston Naming Test. *The Clinical Neuropyschologist, 6,* 334.

Rey, G. J. & Benton, A. E. (1991). Examen de afasia multilingüe. Iowa City: AJA Associates Inc.

Rey, G. J., Feldman, E., Hernandez, D., Levin, B. E., Rivas-Vazquez, R., Nedd, K. J. & Benton, A. L. (2001). Application of the Multilingual Aphasia Examination-Spanish in the evaluation of Hispanic patients post closed-head trauma. *Clinical Neuropsychologist*, *15*, 13-18.

Rey, G. J., Feldman, E., Rivas-Vazquez, R., Levin, B. E. & Benton, A. (1999). Neuropsychological test development and normative data on Hispanics. *Archives of Clinical Neuropsychology*, *14*, 593-601.

Roberts, P. M. (1992, October). Therapy and spontaneous recovery in a bilingual aphasic. Paper presented to the Academy of Aphasia. Toronto, Canada.

Roberts, P. M. (1998a)[8]. Clinical research needs and issues in bilingual aphasia, *Aphasiology*, *12*, 119-130.

Roberts, P. M. (1998b). Bilingual aphasia: some answers and more questions. *Aphasiology*, *12*, 141-146.

Roberts, P. M. (2001). Aphasia assessment and treatment in bilingual and multicultural populations. In: R. Chapey (Ed.). *Language intervention strategies in adult aphasia.* 4th edition (208-232). Baltimore: Lippincott, Williams and Wilkins.

Roberts, P. M. (2007). Aphasia assessment and treatment in bilingual and multicultural populations. In: R. Chapey (Ed.). *Language intervention strategies in adult aphasia.* 5th edition. Baltimore: Lippincott, Williams and Wilkins.

Roberts, P. M. & Bois, M. (1999). Picture name agreement for French-English bilingual adults. *Brain and Cognition, 40,* 238-241.

Roberts, P. M., Code, C. F. S., Hillis, A. E. & McNeil, M. R. (forthcoming). Describing participants in aphasia research : Part 2. Which variables really matter?

Roberts, P. M., Code, C. & McNeil, M. R. (2003). Describing participants in aphasia research: Part 1- audit of current practice. *Aphasiology*, *17*, 911-932.

Roberts, P. M., de la Riva, J. & Rhéaume, A. (1997, May). Effets de l'intervention dans une langue pour l'anomie bilingue. Paper presented to the annual meeting of the Canadian Association of Speech-Language Pathology and Audiology. Toronto.

Roberts, P. M. & Deslauriers, L. (1999). Picture naming of cognate and non-cognate nouns in bilingual aphasia. *Journal of Communication Disorders, 32,* 1-23.

Roberts, P. M. & Doucet, N. (2001, August). Performance des adultes francophones au Boston Naming Test: réponses et variantes. Paper presented at the International Association of Logopedics and Phoniatrics (Association internationale de logopédie et phoniatrie), Montreal.

Roberts, P. M., Garcia, L. J., Desrochers, A. & Hernandez, D. (2002). Performance of proficient bilingual adults on the Boston Naming Test. *Aphasiology*, *16*, 635-645.

Roberts, P. M. & Le Dorze, G. (1994). Semantic verbal fluency in aphasia : A qualitative and quantitative study in test-retest conditions. *Aphasiology, 8*, 569-582.

---

[8] Note that on page 125 of this Forum article, the theories/speculations attributed to Pitres and to Ribot are incorrect. Although this error was detected prior to publication, the rules governing the Forum format in *Aphasiology* did not allow a correction to be made, nor did they allow publication of an "erratum" notice.

Roberts, P. M. & Le Dorze, G. (1997). Semantic organization, strategy use, and productivity in bilingual semantic verbal fluency. *Brain and Language, 59*, 412-449.

Roberts, P. M. & Le Dorze, G. (1998). Bilingual aphasia: semantic organization, strategy use, and productivity in semantic verbal fluency. *Brain and Language, 65*, 287-312.

Roberts, P. M. & Shenker, R. C. (2007). Assessment and treatment of stuttering in bilingual speakers. In: R. F. Curlee, & E. G. Conture (Eds). *Stuttering and related disorders of fluency*, 3rd edition (pp. 183-209). New York: Thieme Medical Publishers.

Roselli, M., Ardila, A., Salvatierra, J., Marquez, M., Matos, L. & Weekes, V. A. (2002). A cross-linguistic comparison of verbal fluency tests. *International Journal of Neuroscience, 112*, 759-776.

Sasanuma, S. & Park, H. S. (1995). Patterns of language deficits in two Korean-Japanese bilingual aphasic patients - A clinical report. In M. Paradis (Ed.), *Aspects of bilingual aphasia* (111-122). Oxford: Pergamon.

Snodgrass, J. G. & Tsivkin, S. (1995). Organization of the bilingual lexicon: categorical versus alphabetic cuing in Russian-English bilinguals. *Journal of Psycholinguistic Research, 24*, 145-163.

Spreen, O. & Strauss, E. (1998). *A compendium of neuropsychological tests: administration, norms, and commentary*, 2nd edition. New York: Oxford University Press.

Steinmetz, H. & Seitz, R. J. (1991). Functional anatomy of language processing: neuroimaging and the problem of individual variability. *Neuropsychologia, 29*, 1149-1161.

Szekely, A., D'Amico, S., Devescovi, A., Federmeier, K., Herron, D., Iyer, G., Jacobsen, T., Arévalo, A. L., Vargha, A. & Bates, E. (2005). Timed action and object naming. *Cortex, 41*, 7-25.

Szekely, A., Jacobsen, T., D'Amico, S., Devescovi, A., Andonova, E., Herron, D., Ching Lu, C., Pechmann, T., Pléh, C., Wicha, N., Federmeier, K., Gerdjikova, I., Gutierrez, G., Hung, D., Hsu, J., Iyer, G., Kohnert, K., Mehotcheva, T., Orozco-Figueroa, A., Tzeng, A., Tzeng, O., Arévalo, A., Vargha, A., Butler, A., Buffington, R. & Bates, E. (2004). A new on-line resource for psycholinguistic studies. *Journal of Memory and Language, 51*, 247-250.

Tallberg, I. M. (2005). The Boston Naming Test in Swedish: Normative data. *Brain and Language, 94*, 19-31.

Thuillard-Colombo, F. & Assal, G. (1992). Boston Naming Test: French-Language adaptation and short forms / Adaptation française du Test de dénomination de Boston- versions abrégées. *European Review of Applied Psychology / Revue Européenne de Psychologie Appliquée, 42*, 67-73.

Tombaugh, T. N. & Hubley, A. M. (1997). The 60-item Boston Naming Test: Norms for cognitively intact adults aged 25 to 88 years. *Journal of Clinical and Experimental Neuropsychology, 19,* 922-932.

Tombaugh, T. N., Kozak, J. & Rees, L. (1999). Normative data stratified by age and education for two measures of verbal fluency: FAS and animal naming. *Archives of Clinical Neuropsychology, 14*, 167-177.

Tsolaki, M., Tsantali, E., Lekka, S., Kiosseoglou, G. & Kazis, A. (2003). Can the *Boston Naming Test* be used as a clinical tool for differential diagnosis in dementia? *Brain and Language, 87*, 185-186.

Van Hell, J. & Dijkstra, T. (2002). Foreign language knowledge can influence native language performance in exclusively native contexts. *Psycholinguistic Bulletin and Review, 9*, 780-789.

Van Lancker Sidtis, D. (2006). Does functional neuroimaging solve the questions of neurolinguistics? *Brain and Language, 98*, 276-290.

Van Wijnendaele, I. & Brysbaert, M. (2002). Visual word recognition in bilinguals: Phonological priming from the second to the first language. *Journal of Experimental Psychology: Human Perception and Performance, 28*, 616-627.

Voyer, D. (2003). Word frequency and laterality effects in lexical decision: Right hemisphere mechanisms. *Brain and Language, 87*, 421-431.

Watamori, T. S. & Sasanuma, S. (1976). The recovery process of a bilingual aphasic. *Journal of Communication Disorders, 9*, 157-166.

Watamori, T. S. & Sasanuma, S. (1978). The recovery processes of two English-Japanese bilingual aphasics. *Brain and Language, 6*, 127-140.

Appendix A: Self-rating of Bilingual Proficiency

When you ask someone to rate their abilities say:

"I want to to rate your (your father's, wife's etc) knowledge of each of their languages. This might be hard to do, but I need to you give me your best estimate.

0 means you/he/she could not do it at all; no knowledge.

1 means very little ability, just a few words here and there, very poor.

7 means like a typical native speaker of that language who only speaks that language. So, 7 does not mean "perfect" mastery, or like an expert (or newscaster or author). It means, like someone with his age and education, who can only speak _____ (name the language).

All these ratings apply to how he talked before the stroke.

How would you rate P's ability to understand what people say in Lx? Ly? Lz?
How would you rate P's ability to say what he wants to say in Lx? Ly? Lz?
How would you rate P's ability to read, to understand what he read in Lx.....
How would you rate P's ability to write (not handwriting, but composing sentences, letters, whatever he had to write) in Lx? Ly? Lz

Often it is helpful to do all 4 questions for one language at a time, but some people seem to find the task easier if they compare the languages as they go through the rating task. These questions can be presented in written form, with the appropriate scale written out, for P's who can read or for their families.

Some patients who cannot understand the numbers, can do the rating task by marking the point along a solid line, with the ends of the line marked or explained verbally as meaning "can't do" and "like a native __ speaker".

In: Aphasia: Symptoms, Diagnosis and Treatment
Editors: G. Ibanescu, S. Pescariu

ISBN: 978-1-60741-288-5
© 2009 Nova Science Publishers, Inc.

Chapter VIII

Imaging Post-Stroke Aphasia

Argye E. Hillis
The Johns Hopkins University School of Medicine,
Baltimore, MD, U.S.A.

A. Contributions to Experimental/ Theoretical Knowledge

Imaging Studies of Aphasia Syndromes

CT Scans. Imaging studies of aphasia began as soon as CT scans of the brain were available to reliably demonstrate the site of lesion in patients following chronic stroke. These early studies largely confirmed lesion/syndrome associations based on earlier autopsy studies. For example, a number of investigators obtained CT scans of patients with Broca's aphasia, characterized by nonfluent, agrammatic speech and writing, better naming of nouns than verbs or function words, impaired speech articulation, spelling impairments, and relatively intact auditory comprehension except for syntactically complex sentences. These patients were often, although not always (see [1]) found to have infarcts involving the distribution of the superior division of the left middle cerebral artery, involving left posterior inferior frontal cortex (including Broca's area, or Brodmann's area, or BA, 44 and 45 [2]; see also [3]). At that time there was a theoretical debate concerning whether or not Broca's Aphasia (or any other aphasia syndrome) was a theoretically coherent syndrome; imaging studies contributed to resolving this issue. The controversy concerned whether or not a single underlying deficit could account for the various features of the syndrome, such as agrammatic speech production and asyntactic comprehension (see [4]; [5] for discussion). Agrammatic speech production refers to telegraphic speech, often devoid of function words such as "the" and "of". Asyntactic comprehension refers to misunderstanding the syntactic structure of sentences, while understanding the content words. For example, a patient may misunderstand the sentence, "The man was kissed by the woman" as "The man kissed the woman." Although some authors believed that these two deficits reflected damage to a single underlying syntactic processing mechanism [4, 6, 7], others argued that impaired production and comprehension were dissociable deficits that frequently co-occur because they are subserved by adjacent brain regions [8-11]. Imaging studies confirmed that small lesions affecting only part of the distribution of the superior division of the left MCA result in only one or two of the clinical features of Broca's aphasia. For example, from CT scan studies it was observed that damage to Broca's area alone resulted in non-fluent, effortful speech with impaired articulation due to impaired motor planning of speech production, but did not result in the entire syndrome of Broca's aphasia [12]. Rather, the complete syndrome of Broca's aphasia, including agrammatic speech and asyntactic comprehension, required a more extensive damage in the distribution of the superior division of the left MCA [12, 13].

Likewise, CT scan studies showed that Wernicke's Aphasia, characterized by fluent, jargon speech with impaired comprehension of both spoken and written words resulted from extensive damage in the territory of the inferior division of the left MCA [2, 14, 15]. More discrete damage affecting only a small part of that distribution was found, mostly with later MRI studies that could reveal smaller lesions, to result in individual components of the syndrome, such as impaired naming [16] or jargon speech with intact comprehension of written words [17]. Transcortical motor aphasia is a syndrome that is very similar to Broca's aphasia, except that the individual is able to repeat fluently and accurately. Evidence from CT studies indicate that transcortical motor aphasia is typically associated with infarcts in the territory of the left anterior cerebral artery (ACA) territory [18] or "watershed" territory between the left ACA and left MCA [19]. "Watershed" territory refers to the borders between two territories, which can become infarcted when there is a drop in blood flow, such that blood does not reach the distal part of the vascular territory. Transcortical sensory aphasia, which is similar to Wernicke's aphasia, except that repetition is preserved, is associated with infarcts in the watershed territory between the left MCA and posterior cerebral artery (PCA) [20], as illustrated by Figure 1. Mixed transcortical aphasia, characterized by preserved repetition, but impairment in all other language functions, is associated with lesions involving both watershed territories between the left ACA and MCA, and between left PCA and MCA, preserving Broca's and Wernicke's area, but cutting these important language areas off from the remainder of the brain [21]. To illustrate, Maeshima, et al. [21] reported a case of mixed transcortical aphasia caused by cerebral embolism. MRI showed left frontal and parieto-occipital infarcts, but single photon emission CT (SPECT) revealed a larger area of hypoperfusion involving all of the left hemisphere except for a portion of the left perisylvian language areas (Broca's and Wernicke's areas). Results were consistent with the hypothesis that mixed transcortical aphasia is due to isolation of perisylvian speech areas, disconnecting them from surrounding areas. This combination of watershed lesions, sometimes referred to as "isolation of the speech area" often occurs when there is a sudden drop in blood pressure, such blood flow is insufficient to reach the distal vascular territories. However, damage from other causes that happens to isolate Broca's and Wernicke's areas from other parts of the brain can also cause Mixed Transcortical Aphasia, as illustrated in Figure 2.

Another well described language syndrome, alexia without agraphia (also called pure alexia or "letter-by-letter reading") is characterized by impaired reading, but preserved recognition of words spelled aloud and preserved writing. Often patients can read very slowly, by naming individual letters, although letter identification is typically at least mildly impaired. Autopsy studies from the 1800's provide evidence that this clinical syndrome is associated with co-occurrence of two lesions – one in the left occipital lobe (causing right homonymous hemianopia) and one in the splenium of the corpus collosum.

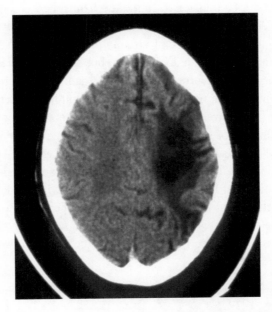

Figure 1. CT scan of a patient with a posterior "watershed" lesion between left PCA and left MCA territory and associated transcortical sensory aphasia (fluent, jargon speech and impaired comprehension, but intact repetition).

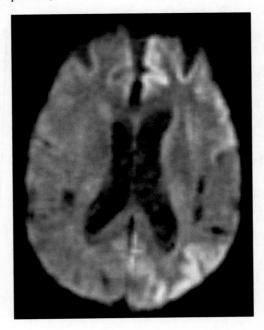

Figure 2. DWI of a patient with mixed transcortical aphasia associated with "isolation of the speech area" associated with subtle cortical signal abnormalities on DWI caused by Creutzfeldt Jakob Disease.

Both of these lesions are caused by occlusion of the left PCA. Dejerine [22] accounted for the syndrome by postulating that the patient would process visual information (printed words) in the right occipital lobe only (because of the lesion in the left occipital lobe), but the visual information could not be transferred to the left hemisphere to be understood or named due to the lesion in the splenium. The same combination of lesions can account for patients with "Optic Aphasia" -- impaired naming of visually presented objects, with intact naming of the same objects to definition or tactile exploration, but some preserved "recognition" of the visual stimulus by performing an appropriate gesture. Again, the deficit is ascribed to the fact that all visual information must be first processed in the right hemisphere but "recognition" of the stimulus cannot be transferred to the left hemisphere to support naming [23]. This lesion/syndrome association for Alexia without Agraphia and Optic Aphasia has been confirmed with CT and MRI scans of patients with alexia without agraphia and/or Optic Aphasia [24-26]. Occasional patients with Alexia without Agraphia (and Optic Aphasia) have had damage to the left occipital lobe and/or fusiform gyrus without damage to the splenium [24]. However, one such patient was found to have hypoperfusion of the splenium, using magnetic resonance perfusion weighted imaging, which reveals dysfunctional as well as structurally damaged tissue [27]; see Figure 3). When the splenium was reperfused, reading and picture naming improved.

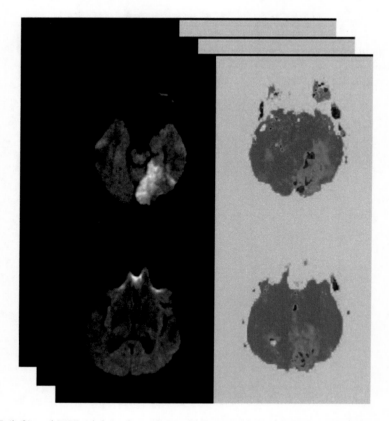

Figure 3. DWI (left) and PWI (right) of a patient with Pure Alexia and Optic Aphasia, associated with infarct in the left occipital lobe, but hypoperfusion of the entire left PCA territory, including the splenium.

Functional Imaging. Post-stroke aphasia syndromes have also been studied using FDG-Positron emission tomography (PET) to determine areas of altered metabolism associated with some task; O^{15} PET, SPECT, or arterial spin labeling perfusion MRI to determined areas of altered blood flow; bolus-tracking PWI to determine areas of altered arrival and clearance of a bolus of contrast (closely related to blood flow); and fMRI to determine areas where a hemodynamic response is temporally linked to an event or task.

For example, PET studies by Metter and colleagues demonstrated that the area of altered cerebral glucose metabolism in aphasic patients consistently extends beyond brain regions that are structurally damaged. In their studies, all right-handed patients with left hemisphere structural lesions and aphasia had altered metabolism in left temporoparietal cortex [28, 29; see 30 for review]. The aphasic patients inconsistently had metabolic abnormalities in undamaged, left prefrontal lobe and thalamus that could account for variations in their clinical deficits.

MRI studies that reveal areas of dysfunctional tissue have largely confirmed the relationships between clinical aphasia syndromes and particular vascular territories as described above. To illustrate, many studies employing only structural imaging studies had led to the conclusion that purely subcortical lesions (particularly lesions in the caudate nucleus) can cause nearly any of the aphasia syndromes described above [1,31; see [32] for review). However, a recent study of patients with left caudate lesions and no cortical damage on structural MRI demonstrated with PWI that the presence of a particular aphasia syndrome could be explained by hypoperfusion in commonly associated cortical vascular territory [33]. For example, Broca's aphasia was observed after left caudate stroke only when there was concomitant hypoperfusion in territory of the superior division of the left MCA, including Broca's area. Likewise, Wernicke's aphasia occurred only in cases with hypoperfusion of Wernicke's area.

Subcortical aphasia

The study of aphasia syndromes in patients with caudate stroke indicates that aphasia after subcortical stroke may be due to cortical dysfunction rather than the subcortical infarct itself. This possibility was also indicated by earlier studies of aphasia following subcortical stroke (identified on CT scan), that demonstrated cortical dysfunction using SPECT [34] or PET [28, 35, 36]. However, it was unclear from these studies whether the cortical dysfunction was secondary to the subcortical lesion (due to loss of input from the subcortical structure to the cortex; i.e., diaschisis) or independent of the subcortical lesion. In the latter case, severe stenosis/plaque of the left MCA could cause both occlusion of a lenticulostriate artery (causing a subcortical infarct) and hypoperfusion of language cortex. In this case, cortical hypoperfusion would not be due to the infarct. A study of patients with aphasia after acute, nonthalamic subcortical stroke who underwent treatment to improve cortical perfusion provided evidence for the latter account. That is, a series of patients with aphasia after infarcts restricted to the subcortical tissue showed hypoperfusion of the left MCA cortex before intervention and showed immediate resolution of the aphasia when blood flow was restored to the cortex (with urgent endarterectomy, internal carotid artery stenting, or induced blood pressure elevation). Reperfusion was demonstrated by PWI before and after treatment [37]. If the aphasia had been due to diaschisis or directly due to the subcortical damage, it would not have resolved with reperfusion of the cortex, since the subcortical infarct was still present after intervention.

Evidence for the neural substrates underlying specific cognitive processes underlying language

So far, we have discussed language deficits primarily in terms of clinical syndromes. As pointed out above, each syndrome is a collection of deficits in relatively independent language functions that depend on areas of the brain that are supplied by a single major artery or branch. For instance, Broca's aphasia includes impaired planning and programming of speech articulation, impaired naming of verbs and functors, and asyntactic comprehension (impaired processing of complex syntactic forms). These component features commonly co-occur not because they have a shared underlying cognitive process, but because they both depend on areas of brain supplied by the anterior division of the left MCA. But there is accumulating evidence that each of these language tasks (e.g., naming of verbs) is also complex, requiring a number of cognitive processes that can be independently disrupted by brain damage. To illustrate, oral naming of a picture of an action (say, "running"), requires: (i) recognizing the picture as a familiar action; (ii) accessing a semantic representation of [running] that distinguishes it from other actions such as [walking] or [swimming]; (iii) accessing a modality-independent lexical representation, or lemma, that specifies its grammatical class; (iv) selecting a particular morphological form ("running" versus run, ran, runs); (v) accessing a modality-specific lexical phonological representation that specifies the learned pronunciation; (vi) accessing motor plans and programs for articulating the phonological form; and (vii) implementing these motor plans with a complex sequence of movements of the jaw, lips, palate, tongue, vocal cords, and respiratory system. These various components of verb naming could each take place in separate regions of the brain, such that an entire network of brain regions is necessary to perform the task. Functional imaging (PET and fMRI) have confirmed that overt naming of pictures results in "activation" in numerous brain regions, predominantly -- but not exclusively -- in the left hemisphere (e.g., [38]; see [39] for review). These regions, including Broca's area and Wernicke's area, overlap with regions of activation during related tasks, such as oral reading or naming verbs associated with aurally presented nouns [40]. Some studies have attempted to identify the neural substrates of individual components of such complex processes, primarily through "subtraction" of activation of a task that involves all of the same components of processing except the one of interest. For example, to identify the area of brain responsible for accessing the lexical phonological representation (the phonological lexicon) for word recognition, Howard and colleagues [41] subtracted activation associated with hearing spoken words presented backwards and saying the word, "crime" from activation associated with word repetition, and found a significant increase in regional cerebral blood flow in left superior and middle temporal gyri [41].

More recent PET studies have identified an area in the left midfusiform gyrus that appears to be engaged in all lexical tasks, irrespective of the modality [42-44]. However, fMRI studies have shown that this region (or an adjacent region) is reliably engaged in prelexical orthographic processing required for reading words or pseudowords [25, 45]. To evaluate these potential roles of left midfusiform gyrus in reading versus naming, we recently carried out a study of reading, naming, and magnetic resonance diffusion weighted imaging (DWI, which is highly sensitive to ischemia within minutes to hours of onset) and perfusion weighted imaging (PWI, which reveals areas of low blood flow corresponding to dysfunction) in a series of 80 patients with acute, let hemisphere stroke. We found that lesions or hypoperfusion in left midfusiform gyrus were associated with acute disruption of oral and written naming, but did not reliably cause impaired reading comprehension [46]. These findings were consistent with the proposal that the left midfusiform gyrus is essential for modality-independent lexical processing, but not essential for reading comprehension. However, the available data from functional imaging showing reliable activation in left midfusiform gyrus during reading and related tasks could be reconciled with the lesion data indicating that damage to this region does not reliably disrupt reading by proposing that either the left or the right midfusiform gyrus is necessary for computing a prelexical location- and font-independent representation of the visual word or pseudoword for reading [46].

Other components of the complex process of naming verbs have also been identified with functional imaging studies or MRI. For example, access to modality-specific lexical representations of verbs, but not nouns, is impaired by acute dysfunction of left, posterior frontal regions shown on DWI and/or PWI [37]. Furthermore, two patients with impaired written naming of verbs (but relatively intact written naming of nouns and oral naming of both nouns and verbs) associated with hypoperfusion of left Broca's area showed recovery of written naming of verbs when blood flow was restored to Broca's area, providing further evidence that this region is critical for accessing orthographic representations of verbs [47]. The proposal that left posterior frontal regions are particularly important for producing verbs (perhaps because verbs require selection of a particular morphological form; e.g., run, runs, running) has been supported by evidence from repetitive transcranial magnetic stimulation (rTMS; 48), as well as PET and lesion studies [49,50].

Planning and orchestrating speech articulation in order to produce names of verbs as well as nouns also seem to depend on Broca's area. In a recent study of 80 patients with acute left hemisphere stroke, hypoperfusion and/or infarction of Broca's area (demonstrated with DWI and PWI within 24 hours of onset) was strongly associated with impaired motor planning and programming of speech articulation (a deficit sometimes known as apraxia of speech) [51]. This study confirmed some earlier CT scan studies indicating that lesions in Broca's area were associated with apraxia of speech [13, 52]. However, this study did not confirm a previous conclusion that lesions involving the left anterior insula cause apraxia of speech [53]. This conclusion was based on the finding among 25 patients with chronic apraxia of speech, the most common (and universal) area of overlap in their lesions on MRI or CT scan was the anterior insula.

However, this result might have resulted from the combined facts that (i) patients with chronic apraxia of speech have large left MCA lesions and (ii) the insula is the most common area of overlap in large left MCA lesions (see [51] for discussion).

As illustrated by the preceding examples, two advantages of MRI over CT for identifying lesions associated with discrete processes are that (i) MRI has much better resolution for identifying small infarcts, which are likely to cause selective deficits, and (ii) MRI can show deficits at the acute stage of stroke, before reorganization or recovery. Although many studies of aphasia have included only patients in the chronic stage of aphasia (6 months or more after stroke), such patients typically have large strokes, since patients with small strokes generally recover quickly. Furthermore, it is often difficult to determine what part of a large lesion is responsible for the residual deficit, since the patient may have undergone substantial recovery and reorganization. As noted above, one method that has commonly been employed to determine the region most likely to be responsible for a chronic deficit is lesion overlap. The assumption is that the area of damage shared by the most patients with the deficit is likely to be responsible for the function that failed to recover. However, this method might simply reveal the area most vulnerable to infarct, since some regions are commonly involved in stroke lesions [54]. For instance, the insula is involved in nearly all infarcts caused by occlusion of the left MCA [55]. As noted, this observation may account for the finding that the insula (or part of the insula) is the area of greatest overlap among patients with chronic apraxia of speech, which only persists in patients with large left MCA strokes. One way to avoid the bias toward identifying areas that are most vulnerable to infarct is to "subtract out" lesions of patients without the deficit. The problem with this method in chronic aphasia is that there is an important risk of "subtracting out" lesions that did cause the deficit of interest, but the deficit resolved before the study. A related method of identifying an area of lesion most strongly associated with a quantified deficit involves a voxel-based approach using SPM [56]. The voxel-based approach allows one to examine the entire brain for lesion/deficit associations, without biasing the results by examining specific regions of interest. However, there are limitations of this methodology as well. For example, if the study includes patients who initially had the deficit of interest after an acute lesion (say, in a particular cluster of voxels) but whose deficit has recovered due to cortical plasticity, the study may underestimate the importance of that cluster of voxels in causing the deficit. This voxel-based approach requires registering the brains of patients to an atlas. This registration allows comparison to functional imaging studies (that typically involve such registration). However, it must be kept in mind that the voxels in one patient may not correspond to the same cytoarchitectural field as the "same" voxels in another patient. This problem cannot be avoided by any region of interest method, either, since the cytoarchitectural fields within specific gyral locations are variable across individuals [57]. Given this variability, it is not clear that voxel-based approaches have a significant advantage over region of interest approaches, except that the former does not require any predetermined hypothesis about what areas may be associated with a deficit. Voxel-based approaches require a large number of patients with and without damage to any area that might be of interest. That is, it is not possible to determine the relationship between any cluster of voxels and a deficit unless there are a substantial number of patients with lesions involving that cluster and a substantial number of patients without lesions involving that cluster (as well as a substantial number of patients showing a wide range of severities of the deficit being studied).

Several recent developed imaging methods can reveal the entire area of dysfunctional tissue, including areas of low blood flow that may contribute to acute language deficits (and perhaps chronic deficits; see [58]. We have noted that abnormalities on PWI (also called dynamic contrast perfusion MRI, or bolus-tracking perfusion MRI), which shows areas of delayed arrival and clearance of a bolus of contrast, have been associated with particular language deficits. This method is particularly useful in acute stroke, since it is acquired in less than two minutes, is not particularly sensitive to motion artifact, and has good spatial resolution over the entire brain. It can be repeated serially over the course of recovery, to determine areas where hypoperfusion is associated with a particular deficit, and where reperfusion results in recovery of the deficit. For example, the patient in Figure 4 had a selective impairment in oral naming of verbs when PWI showed hypoperfusion of left premotor cortex, and showed recovery of oral verb naming when PWI showed restored perfusion of left premotor area, indicating that this region is crucial for oral naming, particularly of verbs.

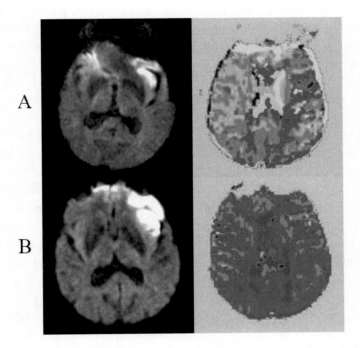

Figure 4. Panel A. DWI (left) and PWI (right) scans of a patient with selective impairment in oral naming of verbs < 24 hours from stroke onset, showing hypoperfusion of left premotor cortex (and infarct involving more inferior and anteriomedial frontal lobe and insula). Panel B. DWI (left) and PWI (right) in the same patient, one day later, when oral verb naming had recovered in association with restored perfusion of left premotor area. Results indicate that the left premotor regions is essential for oral naming, particularly of verbs.

Other methods for demonstrating focal hypoperfusion associated with particular aphasic deficits include arterial spin labeling (ASL) perfusion, CT perfusion, SPECT, and PET. ASL has the advantages that it can show absolute blood flow (whereas PWI shows relative blood flow), and can be used repeatedly to show areas of increased blood flow associated with activation as well as areas of decreased blood flow associated with dysfunction and arterial stenosis. However, it requires more time, is more sensitive to motion artifact than PWI, and loses information in areas of extremely low blood flow. Neither PWI nor ASL involve ionizing radiation; ASL also requires no intravenous injection. ASL has been used to identify areas of hypoperfusion associated with language deficits in patients with dementias [59] and chronic stroke [58]. CT perfusion also measures absolute blood flow, and can be used easily in acute stroke. Currently, most methods of ASL and CT perfusion do not provide whole brain coverage. Nevertheless, they can be useful for quantifying blood flow changes in selected areas that are associated with language performance. A recent study of acute aphasia using CT perfusion [60] is described under contributions to clinical knowledge.

Imaging Mechanisms of Language Recovery after Post-Stroke Aphasia

Among the earliest and longstanding hypotheses about how patients recover from aphasia after stroke is that the intact right hemisphere assumes the functions of the damaged left hemisphere. One observation that provided evidence for this hypothesis is that patients who recover language after extensive strokes in the left hemisphere can show recurrence of aphasia after a second stroke in the right hemisphere, indicating that language functions had been "taken over" by the right hemisphere during recovery [61, 62]. A second line of evidence for this proposal came from sodium amytal injection (Wada testing) of the carotid artery, which temporarily renders much of the ipsilateral hemisphere dysfunctional. Injection of the right carotid in recovered aphasic patients caused re-occurrence of aphasia in some patients, again indicating that language had been assumed by the right [63, 64]. More recently, supportive evidence has come from functional imaging studies (fMRI and PET) that show more right hemisphere activation during language tasks in recovered aphasic patients than in normal subjects [65-71]. Other functional imaging studies reveal activation in non-infarcted regions of the left hemisphere during language tasks that is greater in recovered aphasic patients than normal subjects [72-75]. Together, these studies indicate that both right hemisphere regions (particularly regions homologous to Wernicke's and Broca's areas) and prei-lesional regions of the left hemisphere contribute to reorganization and recovery. What areas assume the functions of the damaged region likely depends on the extent of perisylvian left hemisphere damage, the time since onset of lesion, and the language functions that were affected [76]. It is likely that the right hemisphere is capable of assuming some language functions (e.g., word meaning) more than others (e.g., converting from print to sound to read unfamiliar words). In functional imaging studies of patients with post-stroke aphasia, some of the activation may be related to retrieval effort more than retrieval success [77]. Furthermore, reorganization of structure/function relationships is likely to be dynamic. That is, some language functions may initially be taken over by homologous regions in the right hemisphere and later cross back to perilesional left hemisphere areas. In fact, the highest degree of language recovery is seen in patients who show this transfer of language back to the left hemisphere [78].

However, reorganization is not the only mechanism of aphasia recovery demonstrated with imaging. At least early recovery may reflect restoration of tissue function, through reperfusion of ischemic but non-infarcted regions or through stabilization of ionic balance and membrane integrity. To illustrate, in a series of 80 acute stroke patients, all patients who showed impaired word comprehension at Day 1 and recovered word comprehension at Day 3 to 5 showed initial hypoperfusion of Wernicke's area, followed by reperfusion of this area at Day 3 to 5 [79]. These results confirmed the essential role of Wernicke's area in word comprehension and showed that recovery of word comprehension in the first five days did not occur through reorganization, but only occurred if Wernicke's area was salvaged through restored blood flow. However, later recovery of word comprehension in cases of infarct to Wernicke's area likely occurs through reorganization [65]. Other studies have shown that reperfusion of other left perisylvian regions results in recovery of other language functions in acute stroke [80].

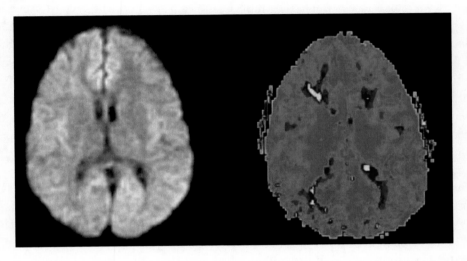

Figure 5. DWI (left) and PWI (right) of a patient with a benign CT scan but profound impairment in reading and naming associated with severe hypoperfusion in bilateral inferior temporal and occipital cortex and frontal cortex, relative to subcortical areas, due to moyamoya syndrome.

B. Contributions to Clinical Knowledge

Diagnosis of the Etiology of Aphasia

Clearly the greatest usefulness of brain imaging in stroke is making an accurate diagnosis to guide appropriate treatment, as reviewed in previous chapters. Imaging reveals the nature of the brain injury (hemorrhage, infarct, hypoperfusion) causing aphasia in individual cases. In some cases, even though the diagnosis may be clear (e.g., a subcortical infarct on CT), the cause of aphasia may not be clear without additional imaging (e.g., associated cortical hypoperfusion revealed by PWI, CT perfusion, SPECT, or PET, as described earlier). In other cases of aphasia the CT or conventional MRI may be relatively benign, but blood flow studies can account for the language deficits.

For example, the patient whose scans are shown in Figure 5 had a benign CT scan, but PWI showed areas of severe hypoperfusion that explained her profound impairment in reading and naming. Cerebral angiogram confirmed the diagnosis of moyamoya syndrome. This patient underwent encephalomyosynagniosis to improve perfusion of the left temporal and occipital regions (confirmed with repeat PWI), which resulted in recovery of reading and naming [81].

Prognosis for Recovery from Aphasia

The above case illustrates that when the lesion seen on CT or structural MRI is smaller than what would be expected for the degree or type of aphasia, some sort of blood flow imaging is warranted to determine the cause of the aphasia. Further, since the severity of aphasia is strongly correlated with the volume of hypoperfusion seen on PWI [47, 82], an aphasia severity score might be used to predict the volume of hypoperfusion. This prediction would make it possible to estimate the degree of "diffusion-perfusion mismatch", or volume of dysfunctional, but potentially salvageable tissue. This concept of calculating a "diffusion-clinical mismatch" to determine the amount of tissue that might be salvaged with reperfusion was evaluated in a recent study of aphasia [83]. First, it was shown that either of two simple, bedside tests of language (oral naming of pictures or word repetition) could be used to predict the volume of hypoperfusion on PWI. The regression equation was used to predict perfusion abnormality with either clinical aphasia score for each patient; then the volume of infarct on DWI for that patient was subtracted, to determine the diffusion-clinical mismatch. It was then demonstrated that larger diffusion-clinical mismatch was associated with better language recovery, consistent with the hypothesis that the volume of diffusion-clinical mismatch was related to the volume of potentially salvageable tissue (in terms of functional recovery). The only patient with a >20% diffusion-clinical mismatch who failed to show language improvement showed no reperfusion on repeat PWI.

Another recent study demonstrated that perfusion CT (P-CT) can reveal the volume of dysfunctional tissue that correlates with aphasia severity [60]. Patients were evaluated with P-CT and language testing within six hours of symptom onset, then serially over one week. In the first six hours, 13/24 patient had deficits in all language domains; all 13 had large areas of hypoperfusion in the left MCA cortex revealed by P-CT. Language scores were associated with hypoperfusion in specific areas within the MCA territory. Furthermore, aphasia improved significantly more when the hypoperfused tissue showed restored blood flow, than when it evolved toward infarct. These results provide additional evidence that changes in aphasia in the acute stage reflect changes in perfusion documented with imaging (and might be used as a substitute for imaging when the latter is not possible).

Treatment

Knowing the location of a stroke or volume of a stroke does not directly guide treatment decisions. However, the combination of DWI and PWI (or the combination of DWI and language testing) can identify which patients might benefit from aggressive intervention to restore blood flow to improve speech or language, as noted above. To illustrate, a patient with sudden onset severe aphasia whose MRI shows a small infarct on DWI but a large area of hypoperfusion in left perisylvian ("language") cortex would likely show improved language if blood flow can be restored to left perisylvian cortex. Such improvements were demonstrated in a series of patients with left subcortical stroke, as noted earlier. Moreover, reperfusion of specific regions of the brain improved specific language functions [84]. In many of these cases, the patients had worsening aphasia over several days, before imaging revealed a large DWI-PWI mismatch, with mismatch territory involving language cortex. Since these patients were not candidates for thrombolyisis days after symptom onset, investigational treatment to restore perfusion was necessary.

Investigation treatment was based on the following reported observations. In ischemic tissue, unlike normal tissue, there is a loss of autoregulation, such that increasing systemic blood pressure results in improved regional blood flow in the ischemic areas of brain [85]. Based on this observation, several groups have studied temporary blood pressure elevation to improve blood flow and function [86-88]. Since this intervention should be most effective in patients with large area of hypoperfusion that is not yet infracted, we conducted a small, randomized trial of pharmacologically induced blood pressure elevation in patients selected on the basis of a large, persistent DWI-PWI mismatch up to one week post onset of symptoms. Since many of these patients had subcortical infarct and cortical hypoperfusion, we measured response to treatment by evaluating cortical function (language skills in patients with left hemisphere stroke, spatial attention in patients with right hemisphere stroke) and repeat PWI. Patients who were randomized to blood pressure elevation showed significantly more improvement on language or spatial attention testing, and greater reductions in volume of hypoperfusion, than patients randomized to conventional management [47]. Even though this study was small, the effect size was large enough to demonstrate a benefit of treatment for improving aphasia or neglect in patients selected on the basis of a large DWI-PWI mismatch up to one week post onset. Results illustrated the potential of perfusion imaging to help select patients for specific interventions to improve aphasia.

Urakawa, et al. [89] reported successful treatment to restore perfusion that resulted in resolution of aphasia and other neurological deficits with local thrombolytic therapy given to a patient 24 hours after onset of left middle cerebral artery (MCA) occlusion. In this patient a Xenon CT cerebral blood flow study revealed hypoperfusion in the left MCA territory, which showed negative cerebrovascular reactivity, while FLAIR only showed only a smaller area of slight hyperintensity in the left frontal white matter. Angiogram revealed left MCA occlusion. Intra-arterial thrombolysis with urokinase, done 24 hours after onset of symptoms resulted in immediate improvement of aphasia and motor symptoms. This study illustrates again how imaging evidence of an area of symptomatic hypoperfusion beyond the infarct is likely to indicate the potential usefulness of restoring blood flow, and may therefore be useful for identifying candidates for specific interventions to improve aphasia.

Functional imaging studies (PET and fMRI) have also been used to evaluate effects of language therapy on degree and location of neural activation measured with these techniques. For example, Thompson and colleagues (e.g. [70] performed fMRI before and after treatment of sentence comprehension deficits in patients with chronic Broca's aphasia. They found increased activation of right hemisphere regions homologous to language cortex (Wernicke's area in all patients, Broca's area in two patients) after treatment, indicating that treatment may have induced reorganization of structure/function relationships. Similarly, Musso and colleagues, [69] demonstrated that treatment of auditory comprehension in patients with

Wernicke's aphasia resulted in improved performance on a test of following spoken directions, that correlated with increased activation in the right hemisphere homologue of Wernicke's area and left precuneous (using PET). Therapy for reading impairment has also been associated with changes in areas of activation on fMRI [90]

C. Future Directions

As new imaging techniques become available, investigators are beginning to combine complementary methods to address questions about brain/behavioral relationships. For example, several groups have combined rTMS with PET or fMRI, to determine if regions of "activation" on functional imaging indicate adaptive or maladaptive neural activity. In some cases in which rTMS is used to suppress neural activity in tissue that showed activation on fMRI, there is actually improvement, rather than reduction, in ability to carry out a language task (indicating that the activation on fMRI did not reflect activity ctitical to the task). For example, Naeser, et al. [91, 92] reported that nonfluent aphasic patients whose scans show activation in the right hemisphere homologue of Broca's area showed improved naming performance after rTMS that suppressed part of this area (BA 44). However, rTMS suppression of the cortex contralateral to stroke can also impair language function (92). Others have used PET to identify areas to target with rTMS or have used PET and TMS together to demonstrate connectivity [93]. The latter is done by applying TMS to an area of interest, and then evaluating the areas where the TMS results in changes in blood flow (inhibitory or excitory connections). This methodology may help identify networks of connected cortical regions underlying specific language functions.

PET studies of particular receptors or transporters, or molecular MRI using markers of plasticity, may also be useful in identifying areas of metabolic changes associated with specific aphasic deficits or associated with reorganization (due to treatment and/or spontaneous recovery). Diffusion Tensor Imaging (DTI) can reveal damage to white matter tracks that may explain deficits due to "disconnection" of cortical regions underlying language. For example, a recent white matter tractography study using DTI demonstrated two white matter tracts connecting Broca's and Wernicke's area, one of which connected these areas via the angular gyrus [94]. The authors argued that the two tracts can account for variations in Conduction aphasia. Another study using voxel-based statistical analyses of DTI showed an asymmetry of the arcuate fasciculus, with higher fractional anisotropy in the left hemisphere, consistent with a role of this tract in language [95]. However, still another DTI study of a patient with mixed transcortical sensory aphasia revealed a lesion in the arcuate fasciculus, a finding that did not support the necessary role of this tract in repetition, as proposed by Geschwind [20], since repetition was intact from the onset of stroke in this patient [96]. Finally, results from DTI in patients with pure alexia are consistent with the hypothesize role of the splenium in transferring visual information from the right occipital lobe to the left inferior temporal cortex in reading [97, 98]. Another recent study showed how DTI fiber tracking and intraoperative cortical stimulation could be used together to delineate subcortical pathways between various cortical regions critical for speech and language [99]. This combination of techniques may be useful clinically (to allow sparing of eloquent regions and their connections during neurosurgery) as well as useful in terms of demonstrating connectivity between brain regions critical for language. These cases illustrate how the study of language and aphasia will be enhanced with DTI and with combined methodologies.

D. Take Home Message

Both structural and functional neuroimaging are rapidly evolving. Neuroimaging has been critical to demonstrating that classic aphasia syndromes arise after stroke because areas of the brain necessary for particular language functions predictably fall in the territory of the same artery. Such syndromes can reflect either permanent damage to the vascular territory or hypoperfusion caused by stenosis or occlusion of the artery. More selective deficits (components of aphasic syndromes) arise when acute damage or hypoperfusion involves only a small part of the vascular territory; or as a result of reorganization after chronic brain damage, such that other components of the aphasia syndrome are assumed by other parts of the brain.

Acknowledgments

The research reported in this chapter from the author's laboratory was supported by as by an NIDCD grant, RO1 DC05375.

References

[1]   Kirk, A; Kertesz, A. Cortical and subcortical aphasias compared. *Aphasiology*, 1994, 8, 65-82.

[2]   Naeser, MA; Hayward, RW. Lesion localization in aphasia with cranial computed tomography and Boston Diagnostic Aphasia Examination. *Neurology*, 1978, 28, 545-551.

[3]   Alexander, MP; Naeser, MA; Palumbo, C. Broca's area aphasia: Aphasia after lesions including frontal opeculum. *Neurology*, 1990, 40, 353-362.

[4]   Zurif, EB. Psycholinguistic interpretations of the aphasias. In: *Biological Perspectives on Language* (D. Caplan, A. R. Lecours, & A. Smith, Eds.), Cambridge, MA: MIT Press. 1984.

[5]   Berndt, RS. Symptom co-occurrence and dissociation in the interpretation of agrammatism. In: *The Cognitive Neuropsychology of Language* (M. Coltheart, G. Sartori, & R. Job, Eds.), New Jersey: Lawrence Erlbaum Associates, 1987.

[6]   Caramazza, A; Zurif, E. Dissociation of algorithmic and heuristic processes in language comprehension. *Brain Lang*, 1976, 3, 572-582.

[7]   Grodzinsky, J. The syntactic characterization of agrammatism. *Cognition*, 1984, 16, 99-120.

[8]   Nespoulous, JL; Dordain, M; Peron, C; et al. Agrammatism in sentence production
      without comprehension deficits: Reduced availability of syntactic structures and/or
      grammatical morphemes? *Brain Lang*, 1988, 33, 273-295.

[9]   Caramazza, A; Hillis, AE. The disruption of sentence production: some dissociations.
      Brain Lang, 1989, 35, 625-650.

[10] Berndt, R; Caramazza, A. How "regular" is sentence compehension in Broca's aphasia?
      It depends on how you select your patients. *Brain Lang*, 1999, 67, 242-247.

[11] Caramazza, A; Capitani, E; Rey, A; et al. Agrammatic Broca's aphasia is not associated
      with a single pattern of coprehension performance. *Brain Lang*, 2001, 76, 158-184.

[12] Mohr, JP. Broca's area and Broca's aphasia. In: *Studies in Neurolinguistics*, vol. 1
      (H. Whitaker, ed), New York: Academic Press, 1976.

[13] Mohr, JP; Pessin, Ms; Finkelstein, S; et al. Broca Aphasia: pathological and clinical.
      Neurology, 1978, 28, 311-324.

[14] Selnes, OA; Niccum, N; Knopman, DS; et al. Recovery of Single Word
      Comprehension: CT-scan Correlates. *Brain Lang*, 1984 21, 72-84.

[15] Alexander, MP. Aphasia: clinical and anatomical aspects. In: *Behavioral Neurology
      and Neuropsychology* (T. E. Feinberg, & M. J. Farah, Eds.), 133-150. New York:
      McGraw Hill, 1977.

[16] Raymer, A; Foundas, AL; Maher, LM; et al. Cognitive neuropsychological analysis and
      neuroanatomical correlates in a case of acute anomia. *Brain Lang*, 1997, 58, 137-156.

[17] Hillis, AE; Boatman, D; Hart, J; et al. Making sense out of jargon: a neurolinguistic and
      computational account of jargon aphasia. *Neurology*, 1999, 53, 1813-1824.

[18] Kumral, E; Bayulkem, G; Evyapan, D; et al. Spectrum of anterior cerebral artery
      territory infarction: clinical and MRI findings. *Eur. J. Neurol.*, 2002, 9, 615-624.

[19] Evrard, S; Woimant, F; Le Coz, P; et al. Watershed cerebral infarcts: retrospective
      study of 24 cases. *Neurol. Res.*, 1992, 14, 97-99.

[20] Geschwind, N. Disconnexion syndromes in animals and man. *Brain*, 1965, 88, 237-
      294, 585-644.

[21] Maeshima, S; Toshiro, H; Sekiguchi, E; et al. Transcortical mixed aphasia due to
      cerebral infarction in left inferior frontal love and temporo-parietal lobe.
      Neuroradiology, 2002, 44, 133-137.

[22] Dejerine, J. Sur un cas de cécité verbale avec agraphie, suivi d'autopsie. *Comptes
      Rendus Hebdomadaires des Séances et Mémoires de la Société de Biologie*. Ninth
      series, 1891, 3, 197-201.

[23] Freund, CS. Über optische Aphasia and Seelenblindheit. *Archiv Psychiatrie und
      Nervenkrankheiten*, 1889, 20, 276-297.

[24] Binder, JR; Mohr, JP. The topography of callosal reading pathways: a case-control
      analysis. *Brain*, 1992, 115, 1807-1826.

[25] Cohen, L; Dehaene, S; Naccache, L; et al. The visual word form area: spatial and
      temporal characterization of an initial stage of reading in normal subjects and posterior
      split-brain patients. *Brain*, 2000, 123, 291-307.

[26] Hillis, AE; Caramazza, A. Cognitive and neural mechanisms underlying visual and
      semantic processing. *J. Cogn. Neurosci.*, 1995, 7, 457-478.

[27] Marshall, RS. Neuroimaging correlates of stroke recovery. Paper presented at the 28th International Stroke Meeting. *Phoenix*, AZ, 2003.

[28] Metter, EJ; Kempler, D; Hanson, WR; et al. Cerebral glucose metabolism: differences in Wernicke's, Broca's and Conduction aphasia. In: *Clinical Aphasiology, vol. 16* (R. H. Brookshire, ed), 97-104. Minneapolis: BRK Publishers, 1986.

[29] Metter, EJ; Wasterlain, CG; Kuhl, DE; et al. FDG positron emission tomography to a study of aphasia. *Ann. Neurol.*, 1983, 10, 173-183.

[30] Metter, EJ. Brain-behavior relationships in aphasia studied by positron emission tomography. *Ann. NY Acad. Sci.*, 1991, 620, 153-164.

[31] Naeser, MA; Alexander, MP; Helms-Estabrook, N; et al. Aphasia with predominantly subcortical lesion sites. *Arch. Neurol.*, 1982, 39, 2-14.

[32] Nadeau, S; Crosson, B. Subcortical aphasia. *Brain Lang*, 1997, 58, 355-402.

[33] Hillis, AE; Barker, PB; Wityk, RJ; et al. Variability in subcortical aphasia is due to variable sites of cortical hypoperfusion. *Brain Lang*, 2004, 89, 524-530.

[34] Vallar, G; Perani, D; Cappa, SF; et al. Recovery of aphasia and neglect after subcortical stroke: neuropsychological and cerebral perfusion study. *J. Neurol. Neurosurg. Psychiatry*, 1988, 51, 1269-1276.

[35] Skyhøj-Olsen, T; Bruhn, P; Oberg, RG. Cortical hypoperfusion as a possible cause of "subcortical aphasia." *Brain*, 1986, 106, 393-410.

[36] Baron, JC; D'Antona, R; Pantano, P; et al. Effects of thalamic stroke on energy metabolism in the cerebral cortex. *Brain*, 1986, 109, 1243-1259.

[37] Hillis, AE; Kane, A; Tuffiash, E; et al. Reperfusion of specific brain regions by raising blood pressure restores selective language functions in subacute stroke. *Brain Lang*, 2002, 79, 495-510.

[38] Warburton, E; Wise, RJS; Price, CJ; et al. Noun and verb retrieval by normal subjects: Studies with PET. *Brain*, 1996, 119, 159-179.

[39] Price, C. An overview of speech comprehension and production. In: *Human Brain Function* (R. S. J. Frackowiak, K. J. Friston, C. D. Frith, R. J. Dolan, C. J. Price, S. Zeki, J. Ashburner, & W. Penny (Eds.)), 517-532. London: Elsevier, 2004.

[40] Peterson, SE; Fox, PT; Posner, MI; et al. Positron emission tomography studies of the cortical anatomy of single word processing. *Nature*, 1988, 331, 585-589.

[41] Howard, D; Patterson, K; Wise, R; et al. The cortical localization of the lexicons. *Brain*, 1992, 115, 1769-1782.

[42] Buchel, C; Raedler, T; Sommer, M; et al. White matter asymmetry in the human brain: a diffusion tensor MRI study. *Cereb Cortex*, 2004, 14, 945-951.

[43] Price, CJ; Devlin, JT. The myth of the visual word form area. *Neuroimage*, 2003, 19, 473-481.

[44] Price, CJ; Winterburn, D; Giraud, AL; et al. Cortical localization of the visual and auditory word form areas: A reconsideration of the evidence. *Brain Lang*, 2003, 86, 272-286.

[45] Cohen, L; Lehericy, S; Chochon, F; et al. Language-specific tuning of visual cortex? Functional properties of the visual word form area. *Brain*, 2002, 125, 1054-1069.

[46] Hillis, AE; Newhart, M; Heidler, J; et al. The roles of the "visual word form area" in reading. *Neuroimage*, 2005, 24, 548-559.

[47] Hillis, AE; Wityk, R; Barker, PB; et al. Neural regions essential for writing verbs. *Nat. Neurosci.*, 2003, 6, 19-20.

[48] Shapiro, KA; Pascual-Leone, A; Mottaghy, FM; et al. Grammatical distinctions in the left frontal cortex. *J. Cogn. Neurosci.*, 2001, 13, 713-720.

[49] Tranel, D; Damasio, H; Damasio, A. On the neurology of naming. In: *Anomia* (H. Goodglass, ed), London: Academic Press, 1997.

[50] Tranel, D; Adolphs, R; Demasio, AR. A neural basis for the retrieval of words for actions. *Cogn. Neuropsych.*, 2001, 18, 655-670.

[51] Hillis, AE; Work, M; Breese, EL; et al. Re-examining the brain regions crucial for orchestrating speech articulation. *Brain*, 2004, 127, 1479-1487.

[52] Schiff, HB; Alexander, MP; Naeser, MA; et al. Aphemia. Clinical-anatomic correlations. *Arch. Neurol.*, 1983, 40, 720-727.

[53] Dronkers, NF. A new brain region for coordinating speech articulation. *Nature*, 1996, 384, 159-161.

[54] Caviness, V; Makris, N; Montinaro, E; et al. Anatomy of stroke, Part I: An MRI-based topographic and volumetric system of analysis. *Stroke*, 2002, 22, 2549-2556.

[55] Finley, A; Saver, J; Alger, J; et al. Diffusion weighted imaging assesment of insular vulnerability in acute middle cerebral artery infarction [abstract]. *Stroke*, 2003, 34, 259.

[56] Bates, E; Wilson, SM; Saygin, AP; et al. Voxel-based lesion-symptom mapping. *Nature Neurosci.*, 2003, 6, 448-450.

[57] Whitaker, HA; Selnes, O. Anatomic variations in the cortex: individual differences and the problem of the localization of language functions. *Ann. NY Acad. Sci.*, 1976 , 280, 844-854.

[58] Love, T; Swinney, D; Wong, E; et al. Perfusion imaging and stroke: A more sensitive measure of the brain bases of cognitive deficits. *Aphasiology*, 2002, 16, 873-883.

[59] Cooke, A; DeVita, C; Gee, J; et al. Neural basis for sentence comprehension deficits in frontotemporal dementia. *Brain Lang*, 2003, 85, 211-221.

[60] Croquelois, A; Wintermark, M; Reichart, M; et al. Aphasia in hyperacute stroke: language follow brain penumbra dynamics. *Ann. Neurol.*, 2003, 54, 321-329.

[61] Nielson, JM. Agnosia, *Apraxia, and Aphasia.* New York: Hoeber, 1946.

[62] Levine, DM; Mohr, JP. Language after bilateral cerebral infarctions: role of the minor hemisphere. *Neurology*, 1979, 29, 927-938.

[63] Kinsbourne, M. The minor cerebral hemisphere as a source of aphasic speech. *Arch. Neurol.*, 1971, 25, 302-306.

[64] Czopf, J. Role of the non-dominant hemisphere in the restitution of speech in aphasia. *Archiv für Psychiatrie und Nervenkrankheiten*, 1972, 216, 162-171.

[65] Weiller, C; Isensee, C; Rijntjes, M; et al. Recovery of Wernicke's aphasia: a positron emission tomographic study. *Ann. Neurol.*, 1995, 37, 723-732.

[66] Ohyama, M; Senda, M; Kitamura, S; et al. Role of the nondominant hemisphere and undamaged area during word repetition in poststroke aphasics. A PET activation study. *Stroke*, 1996, 27, 897-903.

[67] Cappa, SF; Perani, D; Grassi, F; et al. A PET follow-up study of recovery after stroke in acute aphasics. *Brain Lang*, 1997, 56, 55-67.

[68] Thulborn, KR; Carpenter, PA; Just, MA. Plasticity of language-related brain function during recovery from stroke. *Stroke*, 1999, 30, 749-754.

[69] Musso, M; Weiller, C; Kiebel, S; et al. Training-induced brain-plasticity in aphasia. *Brain*, 1999, 122, 1781-1790.

[70] Thompson, CK; Fix, SC; Gitelman, DR; et al. fMRI studies of agrammatic sentence comprehension before and after treatment. *Brain Lang*, 2000, 74, 387-391.

[71] Leff, A; Crinion, J; Scott, S; et al. A physiological change in homotopic cortex following left posterior temporal lobe infarction. *Ann. Neurol.*, 2002, 51, 533-558.

[72] Karbe, H; Kessler, J; Herholz, K; et al. Long-term prognosis of poststroke aphasia studied with positron emission tomography. *Arch. Neurol.*, 1995, 52, 186-190.

[73] Heiss, WD; Kessler, J; Thiel, A; et al. Differential capacity of left and right hemispheric areas for compensation of poststroke aphasia. *Ann. Neurol.*, 1999, 45, 430-438.

[74] Warburton, E; Swinburn, K; Price, CJ; et al. Mechanisms of recovery from aphasia: evidence from positron emission tomographic studies. *J. Neurol. Neurosurg. Psychiatry*, 1999, 66, 155-161.

[75] Thiel, A; Herholz, K; Koyuncu, A; et al. Plasticity of language networks in patients with brain tumors: a positron emission tomography activation study. *Ann. Neurol.*, 2001, 50, 620-629.

[76] Hillis, AE; Wityk, RJ; Barker, PB; et al. Subcortical asphasia and neglect in acute stroke: the role of cortical hypoperfusion. *Brain*, 2002, 125, 1094-1104.

[77] Perani, D; Cappa, SF; Tettamanti, M; et al. A fMRI study of word retrieval in aphasia. *Brain Lang*, 2003, 85, 357-368.

[78] Metter, EJ; Reige, WR; Hanson, WR; et al. Comparisons of metabolic rates, language and memory in subcortical aphasia. *Brain Lang*, 1983, 19, 33-47.

[79] Hillis, AE; Heidler, J. Mechanisms of early aphasia recovery: evidence from MR perfusion imaging. *Aphasiology*, 2002, 16, 885-896.

[80] Hillis, AE; Tuffiash, E; Wityk, RJ; et al. Regions of neural dysfunction associated with impaired naming of actions and objects in acute stroke. *Cogn. Neuropsych.*, 2002, 19, 523-534.

[81] Wityk, R; Hillis, AE; Beauchamp, N; et al. Perfusion-weighted MRI in adult moyamoya syndrome: characteristic patterns and change after surgical intervention: case report. *Neurosurgery*, 2002, 51, 1499-1506.

[82] Hillis, AE; Barker, P; Beauchamp, N; et al. MR perfusion imaging reveals regions of hypoperfusion associated with aphasia and neglect. *Neurology*, 2000, 55, 782-788.

[83] Reineck, L; Agarwal, S; Hillis, AE. The "diffusion-clinical mismatch" predicts early language recovery in acute stroke. *Neurology*, in press.

[84] Hillis, AE; Wityk, RJ; Barker, PB; et al. Change in perfusion in acute nondominant hemisphere stroke may be better estimated by tests of hemispatial neglect than by the NIHSS. *Stroke*, 2003, 34, 2392-2398.

[85] Astrup, J; Symon, L; Branston, NM; et al. Cortical evoked potential and extracellular K+ and H+ at critical levels of brain ischemia. *Stroke*, 1977, 8, 51-57.

[86] Wise, G; Sutter, R; Burkholder, J. The treatment of brain ischemia with vasopressor drugs. *Stroke*, 1972, 3, 135-140.

[87] Rordorf, G; Cramer, SC; Efird JT; et al. Pharmacological elevation of blood pressure in acute stroke. *Stroke*, 1997, 28, 2133-2138.

[88] Rordorf, G; Koroshetz, W; Ezzeddine, MA; et al. A pilot study of drug-induced hypertension for treatment of acute stroke. *Neurology*, 2001, 56, 1210-1213.

[89] Urakawa, M; Ueda, Y; Yamashita, T. Successful local thrombolytic therapy for atherosclerotic middle cerebral artery occlusion 24 hours after onset: case report. No *Shinkei Geka*, 2003, 31, 195-199.

[90] Small, SL; Flores, D; Noll, DC. Grapheme to phoneme conversion in acquired dyslexia: Neurobiological changes accompany therapy. *Brain Lang*, 1997, 60, 127-131.

[91] Naeser, MA; Martin, PI; Baker, EH; et al. Overt propositional in chronic nonfluent aphasia with the dynamic susceptiblity constrast fMRI method. *Neuroimage*, 2004, 22, 29-41.

[92] Naser, MA; Baker, EH; Palumbo, CL; et al. Lesion site patterns in severe, nonverbal aphasia to predict outcome with a computer-assisted treatment program. *Arch. Neurol.*, 1998, 55, 1438-48.

[93] Fox, P; Ingham, R; George, MS; et al. Imaging human intra-cerebral connectivity by PET during TMS. *Neuroreport*, 1997, 8, 2787-2791.

[94] Catani, M; Jones, DK; Fytche, DH. Perisylvian language networks of the human brain. *Ann. Neurol.*, 2005, 57, 8-16.

[95] Buchel, C; Price, C; Friston, K. A multimodal language region in the ventral visual pathway. *Nature*, 1998, 394, 274-277.

[96] Selnes, OA; van Zijl, P; Barker, PB; et al. MR Diffusion Tensor Imaging documented Arcuate Fasciculus lesion in a patient with normal repetition performance. *Aphasiology*, 2002, 16, 897-902.

[97] Molko, N; Cohen, L; Mangin, JF; et al. Visualizing the neural bases of a disconnection syndrome with diffusion tensor imaging. *J. Cogn. Neurosci.*, 2002, 14, 629-36.

[98] Le, TH; Mukherjee, P; Henry, RG; et al. Diffusion tensor imaging with three-dimensional fiber tractography of traumatic axonal shearing injury: an imaging correlate for the posterior callosal "disconnection" syndrome: case report. *Neurosurgery*, 2005, 56, 189.

[99] Henry, RG; Berman, JI; Nagarajan, SS; et al. Subcortical pathways serving cortical language sites: initial experience with diffusion tensor imaging fiber tracking combined with intraoperative language mapping. *Neuroimage*, 2004, 21, 616-622.

Chapter Sources

The following chapters have been previously published:

Chapter 7 was also published in "Speech and Language Disorders in Bilinguals" edited by Alfredo Ardila and Eliane Ramos, Nova Science Publishers. It was submitted for appropriate modifications in an effort to encourage wider dissemination of research.

Chapter 8 was also published in "State-of-the-Art Imaging in Stroke, Volume 2" edited by B. Schaller, Nova Science Publishers. It was submitted for appropriate modifications in an effort to encourage wider dissemination of research.

Index

D

J

K

L

Q

R

W

U

Y

V